UNACCEPTABLE

UNACCEPTABLE

ANOTHER DAY LOST TO LYME DISEASE
A MEMOIR

AMELIA JOHNSON

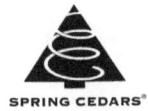

The following is the author's personal story, accurate to the best of her recollection and understanding of facts at the time. Some sequences, names, and identifying characteristics have been changed to protect the privacy of individuals. This work is not a substitute for professional medical advice, diagnosis, or treatment.

Copyright © 2025 by Amelia Johnson

All rights reserved

First edition, 2025

Cover and book design by Amelia Johnson

ISBN 978-1-963117-62-2 (paperback)
ISBN 978-1-963117-63-9 (hardback)
ISBN 978-1-963117-64-6 (ebook)

Published by Spring Cedars
Denver, Colorado
www.springcedars.com

dedicated to the ones who stayed

	PROLOGUE
	PAIN
	FEAR
	SELF
SASKATCHEWAN	
	HELP
JJ	
	BATTLE
WAKESIU	
	COMPLICATED
AJ	
	BEYOND
BASKETBALL	
KRISTIN	
	MISUNDERSTOOD
CHANGE	
SICK	
	EXPLOSION
LOVE	
	BURDEN
NEW YORK	
PITTSBURGH	
	EMPTINESS
TEXAS	
	DEATH
PETE	
	PIECES
DENVER	
UNACCEPTABLE	
	THE END OF ONE CHAPTER
	THE BEGINNING OF ANOTHER
	APPENDIX I
	APPENDIX II
	REFERENCES

PROLOGUE

It was January of 2019 when I finally gave myself permission to take time off work. I let my business license expire, took my website down, and jokingly told everyone around me that I was retiring at thirty-five years old. I didn't think much more of it at the time, but I guess I was a bit burnt out. I felt it in my gut. I *needed* some time off.

Of course, I wonder now if it was intuition.

I spent the first nine months of that newfound retirement doing everything right. I slept well, drank eight glasses of water a day, and ate perfectly curated vegan meals. I practiced yoga daily. I even volunteered at the Humane Society a few days a week, happily walking dogs along the river in the sunshine. And I felt a deep connection to nature as I hiked in the mountains with my husband on weekends, always taking the time to pause and soak my sore feet in a babbling brook, sinking into the serenity of the simple act.

There were many vacations, a total of four weeks playing and floating lazily in different oceans, quality time spent with family, and a deep gratitude for life. It really was a beautiful time—the perfect time for us to get out and explore Hawaii.

It sounded like paradise; I'd always adored all aspects of nature.

2 UNACCEPTABLE

And even though my husband and I traveled a fair amount each year, somehow we'd never been to those islands.

Our plan was to spend two weeks on Maui in celebration of our fourteenth wedding anniversary in October. We were so excited to be going that before we'd even departed, we booked a second trip to Oahu for New Year's as well. We were *that* confident we would love it.

I wanted to walk the beach, snorkel, and swim with the sea turtles. I'd even read that there were a few areas where we might be able to see wild dolphins. I'd planned some epic hikes for us as well, reading all the adventure blogs I could in advance of the trip. I wanted to climb mountains and volcanoes and explore the depths of the jungle—use ropes to scale the slippery slopes, cliff dive, and swim in natural waterfalls. Hawaii was surely an adventurer's dream.

I was itching to tackle the entire Haleakalā Keonehe'ehe'e (Sliding Sands) Trail. The AllTrails app had rated it as "hard" due to an elevation gain of over three thousand feet and a total of twenty-three miles as an out-and-back. Though the real challenge, everyone said, would be the altitude (going from sea level straight up to ten thousand feet where the hike would commence).

I wasn't too concerned about any of that.

I knew temperatures might feel cold, while the UV index would be dangerous, and seeing as there would be less oxygen and no access to water, we'd both have to carry hydration packs. I was prepared for all of that. The only variable I wouldn't be able to assess until we got started was the actual slipperiness of the sliding sand. I didn't want to bite off more than we could chew, but I really, really wanted to do that hike.

We'd decided to stay in one of those big beachfront condo resorts in Kaanapali. It was a multistoried, C-shaped building that wrapped around a perfectly manicured tropical landscape—dotted with aqua-colored pools of all shapes and sizes. When we arrived, I saw that it was gorgeous. The epitome of relaxation. Yet, as I sat reclined on a poolside lounger on our first day there, I struggled not to show that I was antsy.

My husband was always willing to hike for me—not even complaining on the days I got us up before five a.m. on a holiday—but he wasn't exactly thrilled by it either. It was exactly how I felt about lying around that resort.

I was finding it hard to focus on the book I was reading. And sunbathing, just for the sake of sunbathing, was boring me. All I could think about was the eleven-mile jungle hike I had planned for the following day, and the Sliding Sands after that, and the one that had been listed as "forbidden" I couldn't get out of my mind. I must have interrupted my husband a thousand times to talk about all the things I wanted to do, and sitting on a chaise lounge poolside wasn't on that list.

I think we were both a little relieved when it was time for lunch, and I had an excuse to get up and move. So I left my content, sunbathing husband to listen to his podcast in peace, and I headed up to our villa to get some food.

That's when it happened.

I was sitting cross-legged at the dining table, wearing only my bikini, thrilled with the elaborate lunch before me. A vegan burrito bowl, chips and hummus, chocolate-covered macadamia nuts, and, as always, a salted margarita. And I was reflecting on how great it was to be on vacation again, certain it would be one of our best yet. But it happened so fast—before I could even finish that thought or take my first bite.

Electricity shot through my chest.

My eyes widened in shock, and my hand flew to my left breast, clutching at the pain. Clutching at my heart. I knew I had to stay calm, so I took my pulse.

Erratic.

Excruciating pain shot through me again—blinding me, taking my breath away—erasing all awareness except for the single burn that seared across my chest and down my left arm.

Panic washed over me like an icy cold wave despite the warm climate. I was panting aloud, and my whole body had broken out into a sweat. Nothing like this had ever happened to me before, and I couldn't comprehend it. Nor could I comprehend that this was happening on the very first day of our picture-perfect anniversary trip.

I was still clutching at my heart.

I looked around frantically for my phone and realized with dread that I left it with my husband at the pool. In that moment, I knew he would be stretched out blissfully, his eyes closed to the bright sunshine, with no idea what was currently happening to me. He wasn't expecting me back from the villa for an hour, at least.

I wondered if I would still be alive by then.

Another jolt hit me. And another. The pain continued to sear through me, sharp and hot—the electrocutions pulsing rhythmically, and my body vibrating and shuddering in response, as if I were being tased.

I fell out of my chair and toppled onto the tile floor in an awkward heap, convulsing. I could barely think, barely breathe, but I knew I desperately needed help. Anyone, any help. I couldn't allow myself to have a heart attack alone in our holiday villa.

Tears poured down my cheeks, and with one arm still clutched at my chest, I started to crawl clumsily to the door, moaning and whimpering out of my own control.

Jerking. Vibrating. Stumbling. Weeping.

I floundered on my hands and knees, collapsing every few feet, rightening myself, and continuing as I struggled to make it the mere fifteen feet to the door. Certain of my impending death.

When, just as my hand grasped the doorknob, it stopped.

As quickly as the electrocutions had come, they had gone.

PAIN

What happened to me that day in Hawaii will always feel monumental—but only because it was the first time. Not because it was the worst.

The electrocutions have unfortunately continued, as my condition progressively worsened in the subsequent weeks and months since getting home. In fact, my attacks can no longer be measured in minutes at all—my pain is constant now. All day, every day. My life, as I'd once known it, is gone.

There are no more vacations. No more volunteering. I can't hike anymore, practice yoga, push a vacuum, or open a jar. I can't even lift my arms over my head to change shirts or put on a bra. I can barely lift a glass of water to my lips. My pain is so severe that it has consumed me. It has destroyed my every sense of normalcy and my optimistic, happy nature; it now overshadows any other thought or concern, with the exception of my survival.

My ribcage is on fire.

Stabbed between the ribs in the tender and vulnerable intercostal spaces with a large, serrated kitchen knife, it's a sharp, white-hot burn as my sternum slowly cracks. The tip of the knife breaks off deep inside of me, and the resulting pain is a burst of pressure that rips through each of my tissues and organs as the blade buries itself deeper and deeper. A series of lightning bolts then detonates inside my chest, blinding me and dropping me to the ground as I sob and gasp and writhe. I flip on the ground like a fish out of water, convulsing in synchrony with the electricity, as if I'm having a seizure.

There is no book, no television, no conversation that can distract me from what I'm enduring. I am often moaning, and I constantly weep as I slowly migrate my way around the house each day—upstairs, downstairs, from one room to the next. I even occasionally wander out into the garden in what I can only describe as a standing fetal position. Breathing ever so shallowly, dizzy and nauseous. I struggle to think, speak, or listen, but am desperate to find a location or posture to alleviate some of this pain.

I can often be found here, perched awkwardly at my desk, as I can no longer lean back into a chair. The soft touch of even the most luscious velvet fabric lacerates and sends jolts of pain and panic through me. My raw lungs—pink, tender, and exposed—chafe against 60-grit sandpaper with no skeleton or muscles to protect them at all.

I have to be cautious with leaning forward or off to the side, too. Any poor posture only adds pressure to this sharp pain in my solar plexus, and I feel the very tip of my sternum snapping off. And I dread bedtime, as lying down is maybe the worst of it all. My ribcage completely collapses under my weight, plunging me onto that knife blade again. My bare, unprotected lungs are pierced further and further until I finally have to wrench myself up, gasping to escape it.

My body craves rest, I ache with such a perpetual desire, yet I am never awarded it. Sleep like this is nothing more than a hope, nothing more than a delusion.

I'm convinced I will die in the night. My heart is unpredictable; it races spontaneously with violent tachycardia. The odd thump is so severe and sudden that I am shaken from the inside out. At other times, I feel that my heart has paused, actually stopped for a beat or two—rebooting maybe, no different from a computer.

My husband sits up with me now, waiting for me to fall asleep first. I lie on my back in an awkward supine twist, with no pillow for my head. Flat to the mattress, my arms outstretched, and my knees bent and folded off to one side. It's uncomfortable, but oddly, this position allows me to get through the night with a few broken increments of rest—even if only twenty minutes at a time.

This is how I exist now. I don't leave the house; I don't do anything. Since getting back from Hawaii, the only places I've even tried to go are to doctors and a cardiac specialist—yet none have been able to help. The doctors all admit they've never encountered a case quite like mine before. They've never had a patient claim to suffer from electrocutions. To suffer from tasings.

Beyond that, I've struggled to explain it. To anyone, really. To the doctors or even my friends and family. I fear it all sounds unbelievable, and I fear being misunderstood—that they won't, or can't, understand the brutality. I struggle to open up about such an intimate suffering, afraid to let people into that very personal space of crippling fear and traumatic pain. I'm afraid to have to go back to that place myself. There aren't even words substantial enough to describe it.

I regretted not having done my hair or makeup for my most recent appointment—recognizing, still, that it would've been vapid. Though maybe, in some small way, it would've helped me feel a bit more like myself.

I looked down at the bare legs poking out from underneath my hospital gown, which hadn't been shaved even once in the months since returning home from Hawaii. Sock feet, no shoes. There was no part of me that felt like the professional that I was, sitting there like that, vulnerable and exposed. I might have been burning for help, yet I wished I was anywhere else.

I hated this type of attention.

More than anything, I hated asking for help.

I knew my fears were valid and that I was not a crazy person, nor a hypochondriac. In fact, throughout my entire life, I'd always been the type of person who was fairly nonchalant at the doctors' offices—looking for explanations and quick fixes for what were, at the time, a few minor aches and pains. But slowly, it all started to pile up. The quantity and severity of my symptoms. The dismissals from doctors. The frustration and subsequent beginnings of my fear.

I hoped that this doctor would be a better interpreter. One who would be able to see past my very normal uncomfortableness and my colloquial words and somehow not assume I was the same as all the others he'd seen before.

"Does it hurt when I touch here?" doctor-number-four asked, palpating gently, barely touching the skin below my clavicle.

"Not really," I said. "Not any extra, just the normal amount. It's not happening right now."

The doctor frowned at that. "I see. And here?" He slowly, methodically moved his fingers down a bit and to the right, following along the intercostal space of my second rib. "And here?"

"Yes, all of that hurts a bit," I said again, unsure what else I could possibly say. It didn't hurt on the outside where he was touching; it hurt on the *inside*. I was starting to get annoyed that this had been going on for several minutes already, and he still didn't get the distinction. But I didn't allow myself to let that frustration show. Instead, I repeated myself, as I had already done close to ten times in this appointment alone. "The real pain isn't happening right now."

"I see," the doctor said again. Though I could tell he didn't "see" anything at all as he paused and stepped back to look at me with a polite yet patronizing smile that I recognized all too well. "Have you been a little stressed lately? Maybe having a bit of anxiety?"

My blood boiled at the insinuation. It was the same one I was always getting these days: that my weird myriad of symptoms couldn't possibly be real. Anxiety must be the cause. It seemed that even in the midst of another cardiac crisis, I had to convince yet another doctor of my soundness of mind.

Doctor-number-four didn't know me. Not really. He didn't know my history because I was new there—it seemed I was always new there. So, to avoid discrediting myself or feeding into his suspicions that I was indeed a crazy person, I forced myself to explain calmly. "The symptoms preceded the stress. The symptoms are the *cause* of my stress, not the other way around. I think the order of events, cause and effect, is an important distinction."

I tried to keep my face soft in my delivery, with a half smile for good measure, even though my eyes were threatening to betray me with tears and my interlocked fingers were showing the evidence of my stress. My cold hands were clenched together as one. It was useless— the leads stuck all over my chest had wires running to monitors that exposed the full breadth of what lay behind my weak performance. Elevated heart rate. Shallow, unstable breath. High blood pressure. Obviously, I was stressed. I was there for chest pain. Severe, incapacitating chest pain and associated cardiac arrhythmias.

I sat up a little straighter, as if *that* would somehow be convincing. And I tried to follow along with the conversation between doctor and nurse through the sharp stabbing in my chest and the reverberating drum of my own heartbeat that echoed in my ears. But all the while, the typed notes I'd brought with me continued to get crushed in the death grip of my hands.

There wasn't anything normal about this.

Growing up passionately playing sports, I'd experienced plenty of pain before. I'd thrown my whole body into it, and as a result, I was often injured. I was a frequent flyer in the emergency room in those days, always getting an X-ray of something or another.

This severity of pain, however, this type of pain was something entirely different. Yet the doctor sent me home, just like all the other doctors I'd seen before—without any medical care, treatment, or therapy. Only more referrals to specialists who I was sure would tell me I was "fine" and then pass me off to someone else. A wicked cycle, doctor after doctor, when I was very clearly not fine.

In the absence of proper medical care, I've been attempting self-treatment with stretching and physical therapy. I recline myself three times a day on a device I bought off Amazon called The Back Pod. It's supposed to help with costochondritis and Tietze syndrome (inflammation of one or more of the costal cartilages), even though I have no idea if that's indeed what I have. I try ice packs and heating pads, pain relieving balms, and massage. I fall to the floor, twist and contort, and soak in the tub with Epsom salts despite the fact that there's no position in which to lie comfortably. Alternating between sitting and lying, I just pray the warm water will somehow extinguish the fire that consumes me.

Nothing helps—not even a steady dose of painkillers, and at this point, I've certainly tried them all.

I continue to spend most of my time here, alone at my desk, researching online "the potential causes of chest pain" and "how to describe that pain to your doctor." This experience has taught me that words are subjective, having different meanings to different people. Often we can only understand something to the capacity that we have personally experienced it. I need a method of communication that removes any of that subjectivity. A method that can't be argued. Or skewed. Inflated by emotions or accused of dramatics. I need something objective.

Pain scales seem to be the method most universally recognized in the medical field, but I've found they're not all created equal. Some are better or worse than others, with the descriptions all slightly different. It's hard to select just one. So here I am, combining all the various scales for the most thorough compilation of all. And here's what I can say:

On a scale ranging from 0 to 10 (with 0 indicating no pain at all, and the scale ending at 10 with loss of consciousness or even death), I live every minute of every day bouncing between levels 8 and 9.

Intense. Unbearable. Constant, excruciating pain.

And it's no longer limited to my chest.

Six weeks after returning from Maui, my mom and my sister JJ flew in to spend some time with me over Thanksgiving weekend. We were all sitting around in my living room when it happened. The warm glow of the chandelier was sparkling above us, and our conversation was light, warm, and carefree despite my crushing rib pain. A bottle of cabernet sauvignon was open and shared among us. When suddenly, I was electrocuted. In the face.

I screamed as the lightning struck—with piercing pain combusting in both of my ears simultaneously and erupting inwards. It converged deep inside my head and tore over the roof of my mouth, down my throat, and escaped out my tongue and my teeth.

I felt as if a hockey puck had flown straight through the living room window and smashed me in the face. But there was, in fact, no broken window. No hockey puck. There wasn't anything out of the ordinary at all. Nothing had happened—not to anyone else, at least. The pain, the fear, the emergency that I was experiencing were solely inside my own body.

All of my teeth must have just been broken.

Everyone stared at me; shock, confusion, and concern on their faces. Then they all sprung into action at the same time, trying to calm me down.

I was standing in the adjacent kitchen, with no recollection of how I'd gotten myself there, and I held my hands cupped firmly, like a cage hovering in front of my face. Not touching, just hovering, as if I were trying to protect myself from another onslaught.

My sister was in front of me in an instant.

"What's happening?" JJ demanded, concern etched in her voice. Her posture was unusually erect as she stared into my face imploringly. I stared back at her through the cage of my fingers, complete fear consuming me. My already big eyes, as wide as they could possibly go, were quickly welling with tears.

I could sense my mom and my husband were hovering with us there, too, though I couldn't see them in my peripheral. My sole focus clung to my sister's face in front of me—her words, her steadiness—she was my lifeline. I couldn't bring myself to respond, yet somehow I knew I wouldn't have to; my look was communicating everything that was needed in that moment. She was my big sister, but even she had never seen me so afraid before.

"It's okay, keep breathing," she said. "I'm not going to touch you, but I don't know what's going on. You're going to have to let me take a look."

There was a pause as I considered that, and then I lowered my hands and opened my mouth. My breath was ragged and unsteady. My heart still racing. I held my mouth partially open for her and my lips awkwardly back to expose my front teeth. My muscles trembled at these small efforts that no longer felt very small.

"You look totally fine," she concluded, scrutinizing my face and my teeth thoroughly with her eyes. Then those same eyes asked me, and I replied with mine—no words needing to pass between us—my unspoken permission for JJ to step aside and allow inspection from the rest of the family, too.

When Monday morning after that long weekend came—despite a raging blizzard and eighteen inches of fresh snow to navigate—my husband took me, with my chest pain and dental pain, straight in to see the dentist.

My dental history up until that point had been nearly perfect; I'd never needed braces and had only ever had a couple of fillings and one wisdom tooth removed. After a morning spent at the clinic that day, a thorough exam, and some X-rays, that near-perfect dental record remained intact.

There wasn't anything wrong with me.

"Are you stressed?" the dentist asked me. Without waiting for my response, he went on surmising, muttering under his breath to himself that perhaps I'd been grinding my teeth at night—though in the next breath, he admitted my teeth showed no evidence of that at all.

"No," I interrupted. "I don't clench, I don't grind."

I was certain of it.

He immediately glossed over my answer, suggesting I try some over-the-counter medication for sinusitis. He inferred I may even have some capsulitis, inflammation in my TMJ (temporomandibular joint).

It sounded like he was guessing, and I didn't believe him at all. "My jaw doesn't hurt," I told him. "Nor am I congested. The issue, is in my teeth." But he didn't understand. "It's blinding. Electric. The craziest part is that it moves around, like the pain in my ribcage. At times, it'll be all sixteen of my front teeth that throb. While at other times, it's only a single tooth that screams. Sharp and hot. It's always changing."

It was like he didn't hear me as he ignored these descriptions and stood by his initial assessment of TMJD (temporomandibular joint disorder). He told me that TMJD was common and that I needed to be patient; that it might take up to three months to heal. Then he gave me strict instructions to eat only soft foods and wear an over-the-counter mouthguard to sleep, as he sent me home with nothing but a few basic prescriptions.

My body had never reacted well to steroids in the past, so I deliberated for a few days. However, as the searing bursts only increased in prevalence, there was no other option.

I started the prescriptions, and I tried to remain patient.

In January, I woke up to find that my jaw had spontaneously dislocated. I hadn't even previously known that a spontaneous dislocation was possible—yet there I was, standing in my kitchen, confused and trying to figure it all out.

By my calculation, it had been five weeks after getting electrocuted in the face that first time on Thanksgiving weekend and twelve weeks after the electrocutions had started in my chest in Hawaii. Was this now somehow related?

It hurt, but in a different way. This pain was surprisingly not much worse than what I'd already been enduring—by that time, I was fairly used to debilitating, incapacitating pain in my face. The *difference* was that it had become constant, less electrical, and I couldn't comprehend that a part of my body wasn't working.

I had no range of motion. Whether I tried to open or close my jaw, it was futile. My front teeth always remained slightly ajar, one measly centimeter. I could barely fit the tip of my index finger between my front teeth, let alone a spoonful of smoothie into my mouth. My once perfect bite no longer fit together. My teeth no longer occluded. I'd been left with only one single point of contact in my mouth; one molar, the furthest back, made contact with the tooth below.

No other teeth touched, no matter how hard I tried.

My husband and I immediately consulted five of the top dentists in our area, each claiming to specialize in TMJD. It's not that we believed the preliminary generic diagnosis from our family dentist; we just didn't know what else to pursue. Something was very obviously wrong with my jaw.

I was so consumed by my pain that my husband not only had to drive me to these appointments, but he had to speak for me, too. He explained that we thought the dislocation had been caused by a massive muscle spasm in the night, or maybe even the result of my violent writhing with chest pain. Yet neither of us could understand why it had happened on that night, of all nights, when I had taken the prescribed muscle relaxant and slept reasonably well as a result.

Each time, we waited with bated breath for the answer. The solution. Though each dentist, also clearly unsure *why* or *how* this could have possibly happened, instead went on to tell us what they did know. Each one patronizingly gave us the exact same explanation.

We sat in the exam room, with me on the dental chair and my husband in the plastic chair in the corner—the one likely intended for the parents of small children. The room was sterile and always too bright. While the assistant (for some reason always female, always in her twenties, extremely short, and always much too happy) hovered off to one side.

Every clinic was some version of the same thing.

The dentist (for some reason always male, always with a smile a bit too polished and a tone annoyingly confident) held a plastic skull in his hands while he pointed out the different parts of the jaw's anatomy. Painfully, slowly, ever-so-thoroughly, he explained that the TMJ was the joint we used most frequently in the body. It was the most complex joint in the body. It was, in fact, two separate joints within one structure. A coordinated unit allowing for both rotational and translational movement, in which all parts needed to work together in perfect harmony.

We already knew all of that.

I may have been nodding politely as their explanations dragged painfully on, but I was screaming and dying a bit inside the longer they stalled. My excitement and my hope were waning with each passing minute. The great effort it had taken to get me dressed and out of the house turned into another complete waste, as yet another dentist only filled air time to make up for what he didn't know.

As soon as it was possible to interject, my husband, again acting as my voice, explained my symptoms for a second time. A third time. A fourth. But eventually, they all gave us the same skeptical and confused look, and we knew that we'd lost them.

They didn't know how to help me. Not a single one of them could hide their shock when we showed them the before-and-after pictures of my smile. They'd never seen someone's jaw position change so severely overnight.

January became February, and I was left with a pile of useless mouthguards (apparatuses that do nothing to alleviate my pain), a pile of surgical referrals (to surgeons who tell me that oral surgery won't actually help), and dwindling hope.

I now spend my days feeling as though I'm hanging from two meat hooks. Inserted into my mouth and piercing straight up into my TMJ joints, the entire weight of my body hangs limply off of them. My face is being ripped in half.

I suffer a constant, debilitating migraine and struggle not to vomit. Lights, sounds, smells, and movements all send me over the edge. My ears pulse with a double earache and internal bass, my right eye feels like I have a fluff of cashmere caught in it, and my vision has become blurry. I squint through an unknown glare and constantly stare into my own reflection to see if there *is* indeed something lodged within it.

An intense pressure consumes the eye as if it might burst like a crushed grape at any minute, but that pressure is in my skull, too—a bit like when you dive deep into a pool and the weight of the water above compresses your head. Yet the origin of *this* pressure feels internal; my brain is pressing out. And my teeth and my gums burn, even though the right side of my face is cold and numb.

My face hangs slack, as I'm barely able to move my jaw at all. My muscle control is nearly non-existent. I puree all of my food, and I've had to download a text-to-talk app to speak on my behalf. While I can mime some basic needs and responses, I rely on using that app, or text, even with my husband sitting in the same room. And the bulk of my communications at doctors' appointments occurs in the form of my written questions. The act of speaking aloud with my jaw is simply too much for me to bear.

Even smiling, the simple human expression for happiness and sociability, has been taken away from me. My face erupts in twitches, and one of my eyes squints closed in a grimace. And randomly throughout the day, the muscles in my face spasm out of my control—my jaw spontaneously slams shut, and my front teeth crash against each other. It's a legitimate concern that one of these times, my front teeth will snap in half.

But as it is with my chest, the worst is when the pain is electrical. I can't tolerate anything touching my face anymore—not food, nor a toothbrush, not even the air. It seems anything can trigger the attacks. And it's always the exact same pattern. The path of pain is so incredibly specific that each time, I feel I've had some type of torturous anatomy lesson. I hold my face afterward for minutes. Sometimes for hours. Hesitant to check, I'm always expecting to find blood as I pull my trembling hands away.

I was certain things couldn't possibly get any worse when, just last week, I awoke abruptly at midnight. Groggy for only a second, the pain ripped through my stomach for a second time, and I was fully alert.

I gasped in panic, and my eyes flew open. I couldn't sit up.

I half rolled out of bed, clutching at my stomach, and I landed on the floor in a heap. I tried to position myself in a way that would stretch my screaming muscles, but when that didn't help, I feared that the source of my agony was not a muscle at all, but rather an organ. I was clutching my abdomen, after all.

My appendix must have burst.

The pain was excruciatingly sharp and intensely specific in location. I was being stabbed with a burning fireplace poker in my lower right quadrant. Slowly, torturously, inch by inch, the scorching hot metal tip pierced my insides. Flesh was torn, and organs were slayed. All the while, I seared in agony.

Yet somewhere in the deep recesses of my mind, I recognized that this couldn't be true. The attack wasn't originating from the outside. There was no intruder standing overtop of me, a weapon in hand. By then, I'd had enough experience with inexplicable pain to know I wouldn't even have to look. There wouldn't be any physical evidence on the smooth skin of my flat stomach. There wouldn't be any proof of the torture at all. This attack, like all the others I'd endured, had to be coming from within.

Something was inside of me, ripping through my organs.

And it wanted out.

I was paralyzed by the pain, lying awkwardly on the cold, hard floor as tears and sweat started to soak through my sleep shirt. I stared hard at the side of the bed frame, trying to concentrate on my breath, telling myself to think. To focus. I considered calling for help. My husband was in the house with me somewhere, likely still watching TV, and my phone lay only six feet away. But in that moment, they both felt miles away. And while I knew I desperately needed medical attention, I questioned what the doctors could even do for me. With all of my pains, they had yet to help me thus far.

I wondered if this would be the end. My end. And I would die silently there in the dark, sprawled on the hardwood floor in only my T-shirt and panties, unable to breathe enough to even call out for help. But a sudden and unexpected sense of clarity washed over me at that, as I realized that death might not be the worst outcome. I took comfort in that realization, relaxing into the sensations and surrendering to the pain. I ultimately chose not to call for help at all.

Instead, I let it envelop me.

If I did die...this pain, all of this pain, would finally end.

Pain Scale

0 — Pain-free.

Minor Pain: manageable

1 — Occasional twinges. Very light/mild, barely noticeable.
2 — Minor pain. But only aware of it when paying attention.
3 — Pain has become annoying. However, you can get used to it and ignore it most of the time.

Moderate Pain: disrupts normal daily activities

4 — Aware of the pain. Uncomfortable. But if you are deeply involved in an activity, it can still be ignored.
5 — Moderately strong pain. Distracting. It can't be ignored for more than a few minutes, but you can still manage to work or participate in some social activities.
6 — Moderately strong pain that interferes with normal daily activities. Difficulty concentrating. Activity level changes.

Severe Pain: disabling, reduces quality of life, cannot live independently

7 — Unmanageable. Severe pain that dominates your senses and significantly limits your ability to perform normal daily activities or maintain social relationships. Interferes with sleep.
8 — **Intense pain.** Mobility is compromised. Cannot think through the pain. Talking or listening requires great effort. Nausea and dizziness set in.
9 — **Unbearable, excruciating pain.** The pain is no longer localized—the whole body starts sweating. Loss of vision and awareness. Inability to converse. Inability to move. Unsteady breathing. Crying out and/or moaning uncontrollably. Near delirium.
10 — Loss of consciousness. Death.

FEAR

Fuck, the internet is scary.

Shit, I was trying not to swear.

Fuck. Fuck. Fuck.

I'm at my desk again. I'm always at my desk these days, reading about different diseases and terrible, life-changing things. I'm trying to figure out what's wrong with me.

Spontaneous coronary artery dissection (SCAD) seemed to be the only possibility for someone my age, at my level of fitness, to have had a heart attack. But oddly, after the attack in Hawaii, the cardiologist said my heart looked normal.

We thought it might be precordial catch syndrome (which is characterized by knife-like stabbing pain around the heart), but it didn't explain the electricity, the duration of the attacks, or the multiple locations that I was feeling. One specialist was convinced it was a pulmonary embolism until my tests came back negative for that. And pleurisy (inflammation of the tissues that line the lungs and chest cavity) was also considered, but upon closer inspection, ruled out. As was costochondritis.

My new theories are cardiovascular disease, lupus, *and* fibromyalgia.

All three together. Maybe even some rheumatoid arthritis in there, too, as I also have all the symptoms of that.

In addition to the daily electrocutions in my chest and still-dislocated jaw, I now have pain throughout my muscles, joints, and maybe even some of my organs. It's especially sharp in the chest, jaw, abdomen, and back. Then there is the shortness of breath, hair loss, facial rash, anxiety, and headaches. Irregular heartbeats that feel rapid, pounding, *and* fluttering. Muscle spasms, insomnia, sensitivity to light, numbness in my right leg, numb and painful feet, and cold hands. The list of my symptoms just goes on and on; I'm checking off the boxes for so many of these diseases.

But somehow, I have additional symptoms that don't fit at all—and there are still no explanations or solutions for my dislocated jaw. I'm not even sure I'd believe it myself if it wasn't happening to me. Yet here I am.

I've tried everything. We called the clinic again a few weeks ago, hoping to get a referral to another specialist. And to our surprise, the receptionist did take us quite seriously that time.

"If she has chest pain, you have to bring her in immediately," she said to my husband over the phone. "In fact, I have your address on file in front of me, and if you don't get her here within the hour, I'll be required to send an ambulance."

We headed straight in, of course, not sure if we should be annoyed or impressed by her tenacity (or maybe terrified that she knew something about my test results that we didn't).

When we got there, the sense of urgency continued. They immediately rushed me into the back and hooked me up to all the machines again. Cardiac leads were stuck all over my chest as doctors and techs rushed in and out of the room, wheeling different machines behind them—but no one told me a single thing.

Ten, then twenty minutes must have passed before the doctor looked up from her computer screen, and I held my breath in fear, waiting for the bomb that I was sure to drop.

"Your labs look good," she said. "Your echo and EKG were both normal today. Same with your asthma test. And your calcium score from last week was excellent. The only thing I'd like to see is your vitamin D level higher, but otherwise, you look great. Nothing concerning or alarming at all. I hope that's reassuring for you."

I breathed out a deep sigh. I didn't find any of it reassuring, not when I knew not a single one of my symptoms could be explained by "slightly low levels of vitamin D."

She wrote up a few more referrals and sent me next door for more bloodwork. I sat silently while the phlebotomist tied the tourniquet on my right arm and poked me, wiggled and rotated the needle—confused. With only a tiny squirt in the vial, she gave up and tried the other arm. The same routine: the tourniquet, the poke, the wiggle and rotation. More confusion.

"You're cold," she said, blaming me, I guess, and insinuating *that* was the reason for the unsuccessful draw. Then she tried again and again, and I made sure to face away from her and my arm as she did—trying not to think about what they might find (or not find) with these test results. Not sure which scenario would be worse.

Still, I got a bit paler and more faint with each of her attempts. I slumped lower in the chair.

"I'm getting you a heating pad. Stay here," she said, abruptly leaving the room. Returning only a few moments later, she handed me the heating pad for my hands and a paper cup of water. "Drink this."

Five minutes later, we tried again. And the same thing, ten minutes later, yet again.

"Are you anxious?" the phlebotomist asked, clearly annoyed with me.

"No," I said. *Yes*, I thought.

She gave me a look, but she didn't bother responding. Instead, she continued to try my right arm, followed by my left, the sides of both wrists, and the back of both hands. I must have sat with her for forty minutes while she poked me over thirty times, but she never did get a single vial to fill sufficiently for testing.

She sent me home apologizing, perhaps a bit embarrassed that, as a LabCorp phlebotomist who does this every single day, she hadn't been able to draw any blood. However, it also seemed like she was chastising me for not being warm enough, not hydrated enough. She was maybe even accusing my body of shutting down from the stress of it all, and I wondered if that was even possible.

Or was this another symptom, another thing wrong with me?

We walked out of there yet again without any answers, and I could feel my niggling unease was quickly morphing into a crippling panic. A million questions flooded my mind. There were tests I maybe should have asked for—for diagnoses I was too afraid to admit I was even considering. Racing thoughts started to pile one on top of another. I was shadowboxing. Coming undone. I couldn't get my brain to stop.

Of course, it doesn't help my level of anxiety that everything is on hold now. My future appointments and testing alike have all been canceled, leaving me here alone with the internet to try and solve this for myself.

It's been about a month now that the highly contagious COVID-19 coronavirus has been spreading across the globe. The numbers skyrocketed from March to April; in that short amount of time, there were a million confirmed cases and ten thousand deaths. Countries locked down, closed borders, and forced quarantines. The police even started to patrol our streets as we became required by law to shelter in place; forced to remain inside where the constant barrage of news is overwhelming and frightening. We are being inundated by the latest death statistics and images of military lockdowns. Everyone's normal life has been halted; everything is canceled. Our future as a world is unknown. And it's all anyone can talk about.

I avoid the news, and I avoid people. I even had to delete all of my social media platforms just to keep my anxiety levels at bay. I'm desperate to keep it together, push my fear aside, mind over matter and all that—but I keep getting electrocuted, and a life-threatening virus is literally spreading across the globe.

A pandemic, my health, my fear, it feels like everything is spiraling out of control.

I feel like *I'm* spiraling out of control.

I wander the same fifteen steps in my house every day, no longer veering much farther than back and forth from my desk to my bed. And I cry on and off to myself while I spend my days researching symptoms.

I start around three a.m. each day, stumbling over to my desk where I remain. I anxiously read the internet in the same unwashed, ragged sweatpants and hoodie, no bra, and hair askew. I'm fanatical, making lists of possible explanations, I spend every waking minute trying to solve the mystery that is my health.

It's hard to know if all of my fears are warranted or if this panic is simply another one of my symptoms. I've had some mild generalized anxiety in the past, but never anything like this.

I live in a constant state of hyperawareness now—afraid of the symptoms, though also just generally afraid. I constantly get this cold wave of panic that washes over me, and I drop to the floor, all alone and struggling to breathe. I think I'm going to pass out. My hands tremble, and I shiver, simultaneously much too hot and freezing cold. I'm tormented by intrusive thoughts, horrendous visions of my loved ones getting sick or in tragic, gruesome accidents. The images continuously, randomly reinsert themselves in my mind throughout the day.

I need to call my family to quiet these horrors (even if I can't speak). I listen to their familiar voices and allow the steady rhythm to soothe me; I never admit to them why I've called. They've already suggested I'm thinking irrationally, and I suspect mentioning these visions would only discredit the legitimate fears I have about my health. And I definitely have plenty of those.

I've now taken to texting and emailing anyone I can think of. Unsure of where to turn, I'm clearly unraveling, seeking medical opinions from all the non-medical people in my life: my parents, my sister, my husband, random neighbors, and friends. I need to figure out what I should be pursuing next. There must be tests I haven't yet had.

I'm obsessed. Consumed. Unable to stop. Whining, panicking—I can't relax. My brain has found terror, a new gear in which to operate.

It infiltrates my every thought and dictates my every action.

Am I stressed?

Yes, obviously, I'm stressed.

Am I having a mental breakdown?

Maybe. How's one supposed to know exactly what a mental breakdown would feel like?

At this point, the only thing that I *am* certain of is that I'm afraid—afraid of what is happening to me. It is a fear of the unknown, and with all these new symptoms, all this confusion, everything to me is now unknown.

I'm afraid I've done this to myself somehow, that there's something wrong with our home or the air. I even blame my diet and long-term use of contraceptive pills, certain that I must be nutritionally deficient in something.

"My best guess is that when I went off birth control three months ago, it caused the drop in vitamin D, hair loss, and flare in anxiety," I proposed to my doctor via email. But I didn't stop there. "The drop in vitamin D maybe triggered costochondritis, and the stress of it all caused TMJD."

I didn't receive a response; still, I continued.

"It's been over a decade since I've eaten any dairy. How were my calcium levels? I'm afraid the long-term use of the pill would have only further depleted my reserves."

I'm repulsed by this. Convinced that an extreme nutritional deficiency has resulted in my bone loss, I'm nauseated that I accidentally, unknowingly, did this to myself in some misguided attempt to be healthy.

"I think my teeth are disintegrating," I wrote again to my doctor, recalling my disturbing visions of my gums receding so severely that the roots of my front teeth became exposed—and while I gaped horrified at myself in the mirror, my teeth started to fall from my mouth one by one.

"I'm afraid I will need oral surgery, probably multiple surgeries. A complete dental rebuild, in addition to a full jaw replacement."

That is my biggest fear. And when my doctor still didn't respond, I went on to tell that theory via text and email to anyone who would listen: other doctors, dentists, friends, and family alike.

I could sense their judgments in the ensuing silence, the text and email responses I didn't get back. While the few that did respond thought I was overreacting, blowing things out of proportion. As they placated me through their screens of FaceTime and telemedicine, each with the exact same expression of disbelief, I could tell their mild concern was not for my bone loss, but rather for my mental state.

They didn't believe me.

Even my poor husband is struggling to take these theories seriously anymore, and I'm not sure I really blame him. It is possible that I'm losing my mind. I'm tormented by fear, though now also plagued with self-doubt as the skeptical looks and judgmental comments seep into my psyche. I'm questioning everything. Even myself.

With so many fears besieging my mind each day I struggle to know which ones I can trust. Sometimes I find myself going around in circles, and I confuse myself all over again—secretly wondering if it really *is* anxiety at the root of it all.

I've never been one to be this dramatic. But now, having never spent any time thinking about death before, I've become fixated on it. I'm terrified of what is wrong with me. I cannot, do not, accept what the doctors are saying. There is a looming sense of dread in my gut that I can't seem to shake.

Something is horribly wrong.

And no one believes me.

SELF

I've always known exactly who I am.

A Canadian-American of Slavic and Scandinavian descent, I'm exactly fifty percent each of Swedish and Polish. Above average in height for a woman, I stand a touch over five foot nine, am lean and athletically built. A bit too curvy for a size 2, I'm usually a 4—occasionally a 6, as over the years, my weight has fluctuated a bit embarrassingly, a physical representation of the fluctuations I've had with my health. I'm blonde, with my father's nose and my mother's green eyes—rimmed in navy with flecks of gold in the center. And I have a chiseled bone structure that somedays could be considered quite pretty, but on other days, I'm afraid makes me look like a horse.

I am an athlete, or I guess I should say, a former athlete. Still, someone who loves to be active and face a challenge. Both a creative and a creator: an interior designer, an artist, a writer, and a woodworker. I am passionate, with a near neurotically fine attention to detail and an innate sense of when those nuances are finally *right*.

My style is modern and edgy, but above all, it has to be unique.

I am smart but not brilliant, making up for what I lack with hard work. I'm ambitious, driven, and determined. I would describe myself as capable, and in fact, I pride myself on it. I am a doer, and I get things done—undeterred by how difficult they might initially appear. A chronic overachiever and, at times, a perfectionist. Never one to procrastinate and uncomfortable with the thought of burdening someone else, I never ask for help.

It's a good thing I'm a jack-of-all-trades.

At the root of all of these things, however, I am a highly sensitive person. A term originally coined by Dr. Elaine Aron, which refers to not only my heightened emotionality, but also to a deeper central nervous system awareness of my physical and social worlds.

This makes me perceptive, noticing the smallest details that others often miss. Thoughtful, introspective, and intuitive, I'm a bit of an empath. I experience life very deeply, am kind and compassionate, and I love big.

I'm also a happy person, and others have always included in that description friendly and outgoing—and they're not wrong. But because I am sensitive to the energy of others and the environment around me, I tend to be more introverted than extroverted. I desire and value authentic connections, seek out one-on-one conversations over large groups or parties, and I often require silent solitude to later recharge.

I'm not the life of the party, nor have I ever wanted to be.

I'm a people pleaser. Highly non-confrontational, with a strong aversion to drama, I'm malleable. Unfortunately always a bit too concerned with where I fit in and how others might see me, I try to be who they expect me to be, which means there's a slightly different version of myself in each situation.

I don't mean to do it; and of course, it's without any intent to be disingenuous. It's more my subconscious attempt to ensure everyone around me is always comfortable, even if in doing so, I wasn't very comfortable myself. Because it seems I always give the best parts of me to others: my comfort, time, and energy. I put everyone else first. I struggle to take up space, set boundaries, or say no. I get walked on, yet never learn, and I'm often accused of being "too nice."

I'm a dog lover and a tree hugger, and I tend to see the best in the world—the magic of the wilderness, the adventure in life. My life goal has always been pretty simple: I want to do good.

Still I know I can be easily triggered. Taking everything to heart, I'm quick to offend, yet luckily equally quick to forgive. My tone of voice is not always kind. I get defensive, project, and am generally bad at taking criticism, usually needing time alone to reflect, to absorb, and process maturely.

I pretend to be laid-back, when I'm not easygoing at all. I'm excessively analytical, an over-thinker, and a control freak. I neurotically over-research and over-plan most things. I'm a fixer, giving advice when it hasn't been asked of me, and I'm a neat freak, a minimalist overwhelmed by any additional stimuli or clutter. I clean when I'm upset for the exact same reasons I plan and I fix: I need the things around me to be in order because it makes me feel like my life is in order.

I'm impatient yet easily flustered if I'm the one who's being rushed. I like winning more than I should probably admit and am always in some type of imaginary competition, but with whom I'm never sure. I struggle to find balance, not great at doing anything in moderation. I'm either all in or all out. I struggle to slow down, be present, and embrace the moment, and I curse a lot more than I should.

I'm not famous. Not the prettiest, the smartest, or the most successful. I am, overall, resoundingly normal. Humanly complex. I'm both a rule follower and a renegade. Logical, yet a dreamer.

I know exactly who I am.

Although maybe through all this, I should say who I *used* to be; that is, before all of this started. Because lately, with my symptom count continuing to rise every week, it's becoming increasingly harder to recognize myself among all these symptoms—no longer just physical, but I hate to admit, neurocognitive and psychiatric now, too.

It seems like lately everything has changed.

Buried in this mess, I feel like *I* have changed.

It feels like an underlying, vague, and perpetual confusion. Like that feeling of having been woken up from a deep sleep in the middle of the night. You're groggy and confused. You'd been mid-dream, but now you can't quite remember what it was about. You thought you'd heard a noise outside, but now you're second-guessing if that was even real.

Had the noise seeped into your dream somehow?

Or had your dream seeped out into the real world?

I haven't just woken up, though, and it's not the middle of the night—sitting here at my desk, this feeling consumes me all the time now. It's a lingering confusion that I can't seem to escape, a tangled mess of thoughts, dream versus reality, no matter what time of day.

My mind has become a void, a vacuum in space. Thoughts float aimlessly above me in the darkness, but they are without any context or shape. It leaves me with a constant sense of unease, like the world is simply moving too fast. Like I'm forgetting something important or doing something wrong.

I no longer have the cognition to spend hours reading on the internet. Instead, I spend my days here frantically scribbling down notes, tormented, trying to catch one of those single thoughts as it floats around me lackadaisically. It might be something I wanted to research or a thought to write in my journal, yet for some reason, I can never catch it.

It feels like I'm always circling it, writing down things that are *almost* it. I've left a zillion webpages open and waiting for me on my phone, though I may have just as many multi-colored Post-it notes strewn about my desk on which I've hastily scribbled random words. Dark blue, light blue, mint green, and yellow. Scraps of white torn out of notebooks. I've pinned notes to the wall and taped them to my desk—words and sentence fragments, things scratched out, and lists upon lists of symptoms, body locations, exposures, oh goodness. One of them actually says, "Oh goodness," and I can't remember why.

I've become obsessed with finding words. Combing through the dictionary and thesaurus for hours, I'm in a panic to make sense of my own jumbled thoughts. I fill in sentences with adequate words, like fear or pain, but am always left unsettled. I know a better word must exist (the perfect word to encapsulate my thoughts, feelings, and experience), yet I can never find it.

Through the haze, I write like a mad woman; sobbing and unaware of time, my appearance is a bit more disheveled with every month that passes. Consumed by a deep, inexplicable need to be understood and to communicate the magnitude of my new and convoluted situation, I will spend days and weeks on a single thought or symptom. I'm desperate to make sense of my life—see it in black and white. Though I later find that most of what I've written doesn't make any sense at all.

I often retreat to my dark, silent bedroom, wearing sunglasses and earplugs, as I suffer from an intense sensory hypersensitivity that only adds to my disorientation. Normal everyday stimuli are now completely intolerable to me. Even the chime from a cell phone can make me feel as if a thousand televisions surround me, all turned to different channels and cranked up to peak volume.

I'm overwhelmed. The confusion overwhelms me, but the overwhelm only makes me more confused. And my once impressive memory seems to have vanished overnight.

I can no longer remember the things people have told me or what I've told them, and while I have never been absent-minded before, I now can't even remember the most basic of things around the house. I leave the faucets running. I turn the food processor on and walk away (sometimes without its lid, and green juice splatters all over our previously white kitchen).

However, nothing compares to the moments of disorientation when I've gotten lost right here inside this house. I blank out completely, then burst out crying in the kitchen or alone in the hallway, unable to identify it as my own home.

There have even been a few times I've found myself mid-conversation, where I no longer recognized the person I was talking to. I quickly became flustered, a bit embarrassed, also a bit afraid. Sitting on the barstool at my kitchen island, I wondered what, if anything, I'd just told this person. I wondered *who* this person even was.

I stared at her face intently, trying to jog my memory. I tried to take in every detail of her appearance—her outfit, her hair. I looked around the kitchen frantically to ground myself, remembering that if this person was in my home, standing in my kitchen, I must actually know them quite well. Surely, I didn't have to be afraid. But I remained confused as to who they were and why they were there. Perhaps on the verge of dementia in my thirties, it was yet another symptom to add to my growing list.

There was no other explanation for not recognizing my husband's sister.

But at times, I do that now. I go blank. Even occasionally mid-conversation with my husband. While he is speaking and I'm texting back, there's suddenly a fit in my mind as my brain flickers to static, like an old-fashioned television set. The picture and the sound all scramble as my brain loses signal. I hear an inaudible screech, and I see an invisible flash of diagonal zig-zags, light and dark, the chaos of the random dot-pixel pattern.

For a few seconds, I'm lost in it—caught in the nothingness. I don't tell anyone about it, not even him. It's all too much; it's all too weird.

Every noise in the house now alarms me. I'm on constant alert for intruders, gas leaks, fires, or any other dangers that my damaged brain can concoct. I'm suspicious about my environment, potential mold or toxicity in my air or water. I won't use Q-tips or tampons anymore, and I fear that, at this point, there is no cookware that is actually safe. Spam emails haunt me for days, and taping over the cameras on my devices out of the fear that someone is watching, I relentlessly obsess that I've been hacked. I constantly ask my husband to review my junk emails and help me change my passwords. I just don't trust myself to do any of these things by myself anymore.

I have to double- and triple-check everything; my paranoia about the world has now led to clinical behaviors of obsessive-compulsive disorder. I recognize it as ridiculous, yet I can't bring myself to stop. The compulsions consume me. I continually get up in the night to check that the stove is off, the garage door is down, and the doors are locked, and I follow an odd routine to do so. I must methodically touch, push, and jiggle the knobs and handles as I repeatedly check every single one (always in the exact same way and always in the exact same order). If the routine is broken, I have to start again.

I've developed rules about inside clothes versus outside clothes. I wash my hands maniacally after everything I touch (even in the shower), and I sterilize my phone multiple times a day. Actually, I sterilize everything around me multiple times a day. Over and over, in fact, until my husband finally stops me.

The threat of COVID lurking outside doesn't help—even if I never leave the house, I'm still afraid.

A few neighbors have stopped by unannounced through all this, but my health, or rather the loss of it, has become the proverbial elephant in the room. A dark, ominous cloud hangs above my every interaction; people are uncomfortable around me now, and I unconsciously absorb it.

They act as though it would be inappropriate to laugh or be happy in my presence. They look at me in pity. Their eyes watch me as I'm stooped in pain and struggling to function, and I hate every bit of the attention.

I'm not myself—and I think that's been terrifying for all of us. I think seeing me this way forces them to confront their own feelings about the fragility of life. If this can happen to me, someone so young and healthy, it could happen to anyone. Even to them. And I hate that I'm the source that fear.

Normally, I would do everything in my power to put someone at ease, yet through my fog, I struggle to even understand their questions, let alone craft some type of comforting response. And I certainly can't tell them the truth. My situation might be miserable right now, but I can't have them thinking that my personality is, too.

I'm awkwardly silent instead.

Then I overthink after each social encounter, and I hate that I do that even more. I can torture myself for days, reliving conversations that I can't even properly recall, chastising myself for not doing better. So I hide in the house, wishing they'd all just go away. It's simply no longer worth the risk for me to try and be social.

The last straw was the neighbor kid's birthday. I shouldn't have tried to go to the party—not with my chest pain and still-dislocated jaw, let alone the new onset of brain fog and confusion and my anxiety surrounding it all.

I'd even dreaded it all day, never intending to go but feeling obligated. My neighbor kept texting me, begging me to come, and my poor husband was antsy to get out and do something normal for a change. It had been weeks since we'd been outside to breathe fresh air, not since COVID had hit in March. It had been six months since I'd last even been somewhere public, like a grocery store. This would be our first proper attempt at socializing since my first attack in Hawaii last October.

I tried to talk myself through it, knowing I wouldn't have to go very far—the party was only next door. I'd be fine, and surely, we'd be safe from COVID—the party was only next door. I repeated that mantra all day as I got ready.

I bathed and washed my hair, then sat down on the floor in my towel for a while and again on the edge of my bed, where I got lost staring blankly at the wall. I tried on a few outfits, realizing that this was the first time I'd shed my ratty sweatpants and hoodie, and my real clothes no longer fit. My stomach looked bloated, which was unusual for me. My thick hair had thinned; I could see that, now that I'd washed and dried it. I looked older. My skin was a little waxen. And as I returned to sit on the floor, staring into the full-length mirror in our bathroom, I didn't particularly like the reflection that stared back.

By the time I'd applied my mascara, I found I was completely spent; not really sure how an entire day had passed like that, with me just sitting on the bathroom floor. And I realized I was scared to go out. Scared to leave the security of my bedroom and nervous to be around other people. Though at that point, I didn't feel I had much of a choice.

I was in pain, my right leg was suspiciously numb, and I felt weak all over. But highly medicated and determined not to let it show, I leaned heavily on my husband's arm and willed my legs to hold me as I hobbled through the gate and into the backyard next door.

People and kids were everywhere. Music blasted from an unknown source, and wet, swimsuit-clad children ran circles around a bouncy castle and Slip 'N Slide. A few small dogs chased one another, and a kid played with a garden hose, directing the stream precariously near.

Clusters of parents stared at me as we slowly approached—cautious to step around the multitude of toys strewn about, dropped paper plates, and abandoned Solo cups. Their eyes pierced me, and I trembled as my husband helped me over to a table and into a chair, then left to chat with some of the guys at the grill.

I was scared.

I looked different from the last time any of these people had seen me, and I was behaving differently, too. Everyone at the party could see it—I knew it, we all knew it—I was no longer me.

The nausea was already starting to take hold of me, and I was dizzy. I couldn't see straight. I was physically shaking and beginning to sweat through my clothes. We may have been outside, but for me, the walls of claustrophobia were slowly closing in.

My eyes darted from side to side as I looked at the friendly faces all around me, the neighbors and friends who were starting to join me at the table. I couldn't bring myself to explain what I was feeling, not only because my jaw wasn't working, but because I couldn't find the words. I was too distracted by the symptoms, too disoriented to be feeling so awful in this picturesque setting—the sun shining, the drinks flowing, adults socializing, and children happily playing.

It was too much.

Between the stifling heat and music, the screams and zooms of the children, the bursts of raucous laughter, and the many, many layers of conversation floating around me, I was suffocating. Every noise, every movement, was sending my nerves through the blender.

I sat frozen. With my mind going a million miles a minute, I was hyperaware of everything that was happening inside of me and completely unable to follow the conversation occurring right in front of me.

I could simultaneously hear everything and nothing at all.

Missing the cue, and through my broken jaw, I coughed out a weird-sounding laugh, inappropriately, long after the correct time had passed. And then I blanked when the attention was turned to me.

"Hey, how are you?" someone asked. "I haven't seen you in forever."

I stared stunned in return, a deer in the headlights. I was unable to make sense of what they had just asked, let alone piece together a reply. I wondered, a bit embarrassed, if they thought my absence had something to do with my paranoia surrounding COVID, not understanding that something had been wrong with me since long before.

"Do you want a drink?" someone else jumped in.

"Are you not drinking anymore?" said another.

"Are you *ever* going to drink again?"

That final question rang out a bit too loud. The tone was a little snarky—judgmental maybe—at least that's how I took it, as I sensed everyone around us go awkwardly quiet.

I flushed. My brain screamed at me to be normal and reply. I tried to speak, but my tone came out much too sharp, and then my correction was so quiet that no one could understand me. My eyes locked with fear and desperation on my husband. He was only ten feet away, and I was mentally begging him to notice and come speak for me—but he didn't.

I cast my gaze downward, hoping the ladies at my table would just move on to another topic. I reverted to fidgeting with the stupid plastic tablecloth instead. It had a puppy paw print pattern all over it, and I stared hard at it, memorizing it. Allowing the paw prints to fade in and out of my focus, pulse with my dizziness, I willed myself to disappear right into it.

I wasn't acting like myself. I was no longer who I had been, only seven months prior. And I didn't want anyone to have to see me like that. I wanted to leave, *needed* to leave. I needed to be home and safe again in my solitude, where I knew I would be able to sit on the tile of the shower floor, letting the water pour over me as I sobbed inexorably. Alone at last.

Once home, however, my stress response didn't end there.

For weeks after the party, I ruminated on each of the conversations

I'd heard at that table. How I'd sat frozen and blank. How I'd tried unsuccessfully that one time to speak aloud. I painstakingly overanalyzed each one of those moments, and I was humiliated, horrified by my odd behaviors and my deteriorating level of basic intelligence. I felt like such a failure.

Dysregulation of my nervous system, encephalitis, and an increased inter-cranial pressure—I didn't know what any of that meant.

I still don't.

All I know is the constant confusion, the paralyzing fear, and the complete inability to handle life. I know those things intimately. And I know it's impossible to feel safe when I'm always waiting, never knowing when the next electrocution will occur. But beyond that, I have no idea what is happening to me. Or why. I'm bursting at the seams with all that I feel, and my feelings are big. The floodgates open, and, at times, I feel everything—every single thought and emotion is released all at once.

It drowns me.

Everything becomes dark.

And with the waves crashing down all around me, I don't recognize that person flailing, alone, and drowning in the dark. I can't see through the murky dimness or find my way out.

I'm lost.

Unsure *who* I even am anymore.

SASKATCHEWAN

SIX YEARS OLD

I remember being six years old. It was 1989, and the world seemed large to me, even though I hardly knew much about it.

Moose Jaw, Saskatchewan, was home—right in the heart of the Canadian prairies. It was an adorable town with an unusual name, said to have originated from indigenous sources. It was hypothesized that the town had been named for the shape of the river that ran through it (which resembled a moose's jawbone). Or perhaps even from a Cree name that sounded like the English words *moose* and *jaw*, yet actually meant *a warm place by the river*. Either way, as for real-life moose sightings, those were, in fact, quite rare.

It was the fourth largest city in the entire province, though with a population of only thirty-four thousand, that didn't mean much. Moose Jaw was a big fish in a small pond with nothing but wheat fields surrounding it.

It had a quaint downtown, where old brick buildings lined the historic Main Street, not a single one of them taller than four stories. The clock tower and train station sat at the end of Main, where the Canadian Pacific Railway trains regularly passed through. And the river, to which the name referred, was only a kilometer away. Located in the largest of the town parks, Wakamow Valley was a serene place that our family often visited.

With fifteen elementary schools, four high schools, and even a small college, Moose Jaw wasn't tiny. It may have been small enough not to be considered big, yet it was big enough not to be considered small. At least by Saskatchewan standards. It had all the things that one might expect: two movie theaters, a handful of grocery stores and restaurants, and a fairly unattractive, no-frills mall with your basic Canadian stores, like Woolco and SAAN.

What set Moose Jaw apart were the people—kind, down-to-earth, and neighborly. They were always talking about the weather and the crops, and they never hesitated to help each other out. It was known as "The Friendly City" in Canada for a reason. The type of place that if you ever had the misfortune of getting a flat tire along the Trans-Canada or your car stuck in the snow, you could rest assured there'd always be a complete stranger willing to come to your aid. It was that type of place.

The type of place in which it was great to grow up.

We were a family of four: my parents, my older sister, and me. And I saw my dad as the leader of our family. Tall and strong, I felt he could do anything. He was our rock. Calm, steady, and predictable, Dad was reliable in every way. Even down to his appearance.

His closet at home held a collection of perfectly ironed and starched Eddie Bauer golf shirts, all of the exact same thick cotton fabric. All short-sleeved. All in a limited palette of muted earth tones. And every day, regardless of climate, my dad wore Converse sneakers, tall navy socks, pressed blue jeans with a brown leather belt, and one of those Eddie Bauer golf shirts. Always tucked in. Freshly shaven and with his hair neatly combed, I never saw him any other way.

Everybody liked my dad. In addition to being reliable, he was mild-mannered, methodical, and intelligent, with a witty and dry sense of humor and a creative imagination that bordered on goofy. He could always make you laugh, make an adventure out of anything, and his storytelling (whether true or not, we were never really sure) always filled me with wonder and amazement.

He liked to surprise us, too, like the time he brought home the puppy.

The story, as he'd told it, was that he'd met a storekeeper whose family dog had accidentally had puppies, and in broken English, the man had begged my dad to take one home. He'd apparently insisted, not taking no for an answer, and thrust the tiny dog into one of my dad's arms and a large bag of food into the other before my dad could get a word in edgewise.

My dad had always loved animals, so it's fairly safe to assume he'd only resisted halfheartedly—despite how he liked to tell the story. It's quite possible he'd actually received the pup quite willingly, chuckling softly to himself, secretly thrilled to carry back to his truck the little dog and the bag of food three times as big.

Of course, he probably should have asked my mother's opinion first—before walking in the door unannounced with an adorable little puppy that had raised both the eyebrows and the hopes of his two young children. But that's not how my dad operated. And this was in the days before cell phones.

We were lucky that Mom was easygoing. A pretty and petite woman with soft, shiny blonde hair and only minimal makeup, her look was simple and modest yet always classy. She wore a complementary color palette to my dad's earth tones, preferring colors like navy and ivory, and was rarely seen without a single strand of pearls around her neck. But even though our parents both dressed tidy and proper, neither our family nor our home was ever stuffy. And despite the additional work a puppy would inevitably make for her, Mom did acquiesce quite quickly, telling us she just couldn't bring herself to disappoint our adorable little faces. And just like that, the scruffy little terrier mix became a part of the Johnson family.

I named her Trampzina, though we called her Tramp for short as *Lady and the Tramp* was my favorite story at the time. But that little dog often gave us a scare, running away every couple of weeks to chase a jackrabbit or gopher, and Tramp turned out to be an awful name to yell at the top of our lungs while we walked around our suburban streets searching for her.

Still, it remained. As my loving and supportive parents were, each in their own way, fairly laid-back, they never said a word about the questionable name I had chosen. And Tramp always returned home after her little adventures away. We never had to worry too much about any of that.

Our parents always made sure to keep things fun for us. Like our mom often drove us to and from school instead of sending us on the bus, saying she enjoyed the extra time spent together. She liked to crank the stereo so we could all sing loudly to songs like "Islands in the Stream," "Eye of the Tiger," and "Girls Just Want To Have Fun." And we often continued to sing and dance in our living room once home, my mother's arms floating freely up in the air above her, eyes closed as she swayed to the music.

She was our Energizer Bunny—enthusiastic, energetic, excitable even—she had a real joie de vivre. But she was also the sweetest person, a natural caregiver, compassionate and warm. She doted on us daily, plaiting our hair in intricate French braids and dressing us up in cute outfits. She was always telling us how pretty and smart we were and how much she and Dad loved us. Mom had this way of making us feel special—like the time she crimped my hair and dressed me in a white fur jacket, telling me with adoration in her voice that I looked like a movie star. I honestly believed her.

Our parents were our biggest cheerleaders, never missing one of our events and always volunteering to help out at our school. And because of them, our childhood was simple and perfect. Even the weather didn't bother us, and winters in Saskatchewan could be especially cold.

Temperatures were always below freezing—regularly minus twenty, thirty, or even forty degrees Celsius. At times, with the windchill, it would even dip into the negative fifties, making Saskatchewan the coldest place on the planet. And the winters were long, stretching on for more than half of the year, while the individual days themselves were incredibly short. We had only eight hours of daylight in our permanently frozen world. But I had no complaints.

I loved building snowmen and snow forts; I was always building something. I loved skating on the plethora of rinks that were found in each of the town parks; this was Canada, after all, and every neighborhood park had to have an outdoor rink. It was as much of a staple as a swing set or slide. But there was nothing better than lying out on the snow in our backyard amid my latest snow fort creation. Flat on my back with my snowsuit protecting me from the elements, I stared up in awe at the dark sky alight with the dancing colors of the northern lights. I wasn't bothered by the brutal cold, the long winters, or the short days. I was captivated by it all.

And come summer, I'd fall in love with that season even more.

Lasting only a few short months, summer gifted us with an additional nine hours of sunlight each day. And those extra-long, seventeen-hour days allowed us to soak up every minute of its beauty and warmth.

The days were hot, into the thirties and occasionally reaching forty degrees Celsius (which I'd sometimes hear people say was over a hundred degrees Fahrenheit). The parks were green, the outdoor hockey rinks temporarily forgotten, and the surrounding farmers' fields blossomed into a patchwork of vibrant blocks of color. Yellow canola, blue flax, and a million shades of green. And with no hills in sight and no skyscrapers to block the view, Saskatchewan truly was the "Land of Living Skies." Each evening enacted a magnificent 360-degree display, taking hours to fade from blue to purple to pink to gold. So slow and gradual, the changes were nearly imperceptible.

We played outside at every opportunity, climbing the big weeping birch tree in our front yard and visiting different playgrounds and parks. But the best part of summer, by far, was that we would head out as a family anytime the weather was hot, the winds were mild, and we'd all deemed it to be "a good lake day."

The lake was our favorite.

Moose Jaw may have rarely had moose, but Buffalo Pound Lake did, in fact, have bison. It was neat to see them grazing the pastured hillsides as we cruised the narrow yet long waters of the flooded river valley on our family bowrider boat. They were always there, in the distance, dark giant forms spectating as we spent hours swimming and practicing our dives and cannonballs in the calm, cool waters. Those bison watched us even as we all took turns waterskiing and being pulled on the tube.

If that wasn't enough, our other forms of entertainment out there included the Canadian Forces Snowbirds, a military aerobatic flight team that often practiced in the skies above the lake. Flying and barrel-rolling above us in flawless formation, we lay on the sundeck and stared up at the planes in awe, watching what felt like our very own private performance.

After hours of this, we could always count on Mom to take care of us. She never once forgot to pack a cooler of delicious food for lunch, a few pops, and our favorite lake cake—a homemade cinnamon rhubarb loaf with a sugar crumble on top. And as we all happily ate our chips and sandwiches, Mom never missed the fleeting opportunity of our stillness to diligently re-slather us all with sunscreen.

Dad loved that lake cake, but he resisted the sunscreen and often burned. Fed up with this, my mom slapped her greasy sunscreen-filled hand on the center of his bare chest one day, and he laughed and yelped as he jumped away. He sunburned a perfectly white handprint into his chest that day, my mother's hand overtop of his heart. A beautiful symbol of her loving playfulness and a lasting lesson of the benefits of sunscreen.

Our family laughed at that handprint for a week.

My mother's sister, our Aunt Teasee, often joined us for these adventures. She was young and fun and always entertained us with stories about her travels to exotic places like Mexico and Hawaii (places we couldn't yet identify on a map). She took us to the Wild Animal Park—Moose Jaw's own little zoo—and for walks along Spring Creek where we would pick cattails and pussy willows. And Teasee had a cabin out at Buffalo Pound Lake, where my sister JJ and I would sometimes get to sleep over.

Kyle would get to come, too, though his sweet baby sister Kristin was still too young to join us. They were our cousins—my mother's youngest sister Mary's kids—but we spent so much time together that we'd always been more than that.

We were like siblings.

We were best friends.

We played dress-up and loved playgrounds, Legos, Barbies, and Hot Wheels, each always trying to accommodate the other with their obvious gender-specific activity of choice. We swam at the Nat and made up games like gophers. There were many adventures in Besant, where we waded in the creek and learned to catch frogs. Big family picnics in Wakamow, where the whole family played kickball—always laughing the hardest when Uncle Ron carried us around like a superhero, one child on each of his shoulders. And out at Teasee's cabin, in the winter, we snowmobiled across the frozen lake and through the drifts of pure white snow. While in the summer, we went to the pool and to the beach at the Provincial Park.

It was an idyllic summer's day, not unlike any of the others that had come before, when the three of us playing out in the yard in front of Teasee's cabin discovered I had a bug caught behind my right ear. I didn't know how long it had been there prior to noticing it, and I wasn't particularly concerned about it, either—yet everyone else halted at its discovery.

It was buried deep underneath my skin and not letting go.

Teasee called this bug a tick and immediately ushered us inside the little cabin. It was a rustic two-story abode that, even though it was 1989, was still decorated in the style of the '70s: wood-paneled walls and cabinetry, and curtains in a floral print of white, brown, and orange. I was told to sit by myself on the brown velvet sofa. Teasee fetched the Vaseline, and JJ and Kyle hovered nearby, watching as Teasee proceeded to smear big gobs behind my right ear. And then everyone stared, watching me intently, as absolutely nothing remarkable happened.

Teasee rushed upstairs without saying a word, returning only a moment later with a pair of tweezers from her overnight bag. She used those tweezers to poke at me for a while, but I guess that didn't prove successful either because, eventually, she lit a match. JJ and Kyle both took a big step back. Their eyes, as big as saucers, caused me to freeze in place; I was afraid to move a single muscle. And as Teasee confirmed I should hold very, very still, she steadily brought the burning match up to my head. A tiny trail of smoke was just barely visible in the air beside me.

And then it was over.

The tick had been removed and discarded, and we were allowed to go outside and resume our play again. It had been anticlimactic overall, a non-event. And none of us would ever think of it again—until three decades later.

It simply wasn't a big deal.

Lyme disease didn't exist on the Canadian prairies.

HELP

It's only a theory. When I think about it, it might not even be a good one at that, as I've learned there's very little consensus surrounding it. No agreed-upon playbook. No standardized protocol for either diagnosing or treating chronic Lyme.

After that disastrous party at my neighbor's, we looked into it.

Most patients take long-term antibiotics. Some do it orally, others intravenously. Depending on the exact combination of infections that one might have, protocols can be customized to suit an individual patient's needs.

Alternative treatments exist as well—things like acupuncture, chiropractic, hyperbaric oxygen, ozone, bee venom, heat shock protein therapy, prolotherapy, and rife machines. Even a gadget called The Zapper was recommended to me, which is literally supposed to "zap" your infection.

I'd initially hoped that all of these options meant it would be easy for me to treat Lyme (if that is, in fact, what I have). But I quickly learned, while there might be an abundance of options out there, none of them are great. They're basically all experimental and non-FDA-approved. Stupid expensive, not covered at all by insurance. And not a single one is guaranteed to work.

So why would I even consider treating for Lyme? When testing is completely inaccurate and the disease is only the theory of one man—some guy my husband found on the internet, who talked to us via telemedicine from a poorly run clinic in a nondescript office downtown.

There are no shortages of other theories out there.

A pulled muscle. GERD. Plantar fasciitis. Is one of those theories better? I've been encouraged to be vegan and equally encouraged not to be vegan. Told to take extra vitamins and also told that the vitamins could be what's causing my issues. There's been talk of mold illness, as well as the effects of altitude. I've been told that I'm "not believing enough" to heal, that I should contact a shaman, and I really need to stop using the microwave. Maybe *that's* the solution.

My weight, my nutrition, and my choices have all been questioned. This theory of Lyme disease has been questioned. It's been overwhelming, to say the least, all those theories, all those voices in my head.

It was the start of May, and yet another month was passing me by, still without bringing any relief. My jaw remained dislocated, I was still getting electrocuted daily, and I felt like I was losing my mind. At my wit's end, my husband and I ended up calling my sister JJ up in Canada.

"I can't do it anymore," I said to them both, forcing out the only mumbled words I would dare speak aloud that entire day. I couldn't research any more symptoms, any more theories, or any more doctors—I was done. Suffocating under a mountain of pain and my life completely out of control, I felt like I'd reached my limit.

They protested, immediately placating and soothing, but there was nothing left in me to give. I felt clear on what theories and associated treatments *weren't* right for me; but the harder part, I realized, was to figure out what *was*. So I handed the phone off to my husband as I flopped back on the bed dramatically, closing my eyes to shut it all out. Listening as my husband and sister had to awkwardly continue the call without me, I refused to speak another painful word.

The two of them dove into reading and research in the days after that. They made lists, sent articles back and forth, and discussed every symptom, every fear, every possible disease, and every treatment option with me over phone and email. They were showing me I wasn't alone. And they soon agreed there were too many theories for us to contend with, most of which were unfathomable. It was exactly as I'd feared. Exactly as I'd already told them. It was both hopeless and completely overwhelming—but in a way, it was also an important realization.

There wasn't going to be a single clear path forward.

So how would we choose? Which theory would we follow?

I would have to try a bit of it all—like a shotgun approach. It was my only option.

We decided I would follow a combination of both Western and alternative medicines. I would treat holistically and not just symptomatically, with a team of entirely new doctors; attacking this from a few different angles. I'd take antibiotics for Lyme, for both my body and my jaw (even if begrudgingly with the Lyme-guy from the poorly run clinic in the nondescript office downtown). We had to determine if that theory could indeed be correct. There would be ongoing research and continual testing through allopathic medicine, just to be safe. Weekly therapy online with a psychiatrist, and testing and supplements according to a new naturopathic plan, too. And with my new team's support and a plan in place, I happily left my dinosaur of a cardiologist, rheumatologist, other general practitioners, and dentists behind.

My first in-person appointment with the Lyme-guy wasn't at all what we expected. Not that I'd even been aware that I had any preconceived notions going into that first meeting, but once there, I knew for certain it wasn't that.

We all hid behind our masks, unable to see each other's faces or expressions. And without any preamble or pleasantries, the Lyme-guy, apparently not much of a talker, had me move from the chair in which I'd been sitting to lying on an exam table.

My husband followed us over there on instinct and stood beside me at that table in support, when the Lyme-guy looked up at him startled—as if noticing for the first time that my husband was even there. "You can't be here," the Lyme-guy snapped. "This testing will require all of my focus, and I can't have anyone speaking to me through it or even watching."

"Oh. I'm sorry," my husband replied on instinct, flustered by the Lyme-guy's intensity. Casting a worried glance at me, he retreated to the guest chairs and sat. And as he angled his body away from us, I could tell he was trying to give the air he wouldn't be paying us any attention, but that he was actually on high alert. The Lyme-guy had already started with only the briefest of explanations.

Rambling off terms I didn't understand, like "Autonomic Response Testing" and "muscle testing," the Lyme-guy told me he would be reading my body's stress reactions to the unique electromagnetic frequencies of different pathogens. His goal was to prescribe an appropriate first protocol. And although I didn't know what any of that meant or how he would achieve it, I didn't bother responding. Not only did I rarely use my voice anymore, he'd just told us we weren't *supposed* to talk. So instead, I stared up at the dingy ceiling tiles, wondering what I'd gotten myself into.

I tried not to move or distract him. I tried my absolute best to focus on relaxing my body, clearing my mind, and concentrating on the areas that needed the most healing. With absolutely no idea if my mental engagement would help his testing or not, I tried to believe in the process. Weird as it was.

Five minutes ticked by. And then ten.

"I appreciate your openness," the Lyme-guy blurted out randomly. "I understand this is likely odd to you, but it can be quite effective. In fact, I'd like to do this every four weeks."

His statement had been directed at the both of us, I thought—perhaps his attempt at smoothing some of the earlier tension. I really wasn't sure though, so I stayed silent. We both did. Thinking it funny that even the Lyme-guy had admitted this was weird, I just kept staring at those ceiling tiles. My focus never broke as I allowed the Lyme-guy to do, well, whatever it was that he was doing.

Standing at my shoulder beside the exam table on which I lay, he methodically removed tiny glass vials from oversized cases. While an assistant silently entered the room and stood further down my body, resting her hand gently on my thigh.

Each case must have held fifty little vials or more, and though I avoided watching the Lyme-guy directly, I could sense as he continued to remove them one at a time with care. In one hand, he then hovered the vials in various places overtop of my body—my head, my chest, my abdomen—all the while his other hand rested firmly on his assistant's arm.

She attempted to hold still through all this, yet as they worked together in tandem, I noticed a subtle little dance started to occur. I sensed her arm occasionally collapse under the gentle pressure of his. The vial in question was moved around with more enthusiasm after that. And occasionally, crystals were brought out and placed onto the table around me as well.

Everyone was perfectly silent, their movements subtle; it was nearly hypnotic. When after another ten minutes, the Lyme-guy softly touched me, and I startled. That brief trace of human connection breaking my concentration and pulling me from my reverie, I looked up at him on instinct. My breath caught. I flushed.

I hadn't meant to gape at the mystery man while he worked, but at that touch, I'd prayed there was a magical power within his hands.

Desperate for them to heal me, desperate to believe in it, I forced myself to turn away from the guy—ostensibly an expert, though barely older than I was. I stared again at the ceiling tiles and the vent with the long strand of dust, billowing slightly in the air. I tried to re-enter my meditation once more, attempting to ignore the large crystal that now sat on the table beside my head.

It was only when the testing was completed that I allowed my focus to shift away from those dingy ceiling tiles and up to the Lyme-guy's face—velvety bronze skin and calm eyes as dark as black coffee. My big green eyes were wide with fear as I studied him imploringly. Now unabashedly, my gaze was locked onto his.

This guy held the answers; this guy knew my future.

Well? I thought, unable to use my jaw and asking him only with my stare. *What do you think?*

Every fourth Friday now, the Lyme-guy prescribes about a dozen unique medications. And after our appointment involving the same, very weird muscle testing, my husband must spend a few hours making calls and driving to specialty pharmacies to acquire them. Shortages and shipping issues due to the pandemic only compound our stress.

I'm two months into this treatment, and I fear every time that I won't be able to get what I need to start the next month's protocol by Monday, and that any delay in obtaining the drugs could potentially hinder my progress. I want to do this all perfectly, follow the Lyme-guy's instructions precisely to maximize my chance of success.

I *need* to do this all perfectly.

I take his medications six times a day. It is a combination of pharmaceutical antibiotics, supplements, high-dose vitamins, and herbal and homeopathic meds. The goal is to fight not only the theoretical Lyme bacteria but also any secondary opportunistic infections that my body might be harboring—things like viruses, fungus, mold, and parasites. All the while we must support my immune system, my gastrointestinal tract, organs like my heart, kidneys, and liver.

Some of the meds need to be taken on an empty stomach, while others need to be with food. Most are taken every day, though some get pulsed for four days in a row, followed by three days off. Some are in pill form, others are liquid. I have to avoid the sun and watch out for hidden sources of alcohol, magnesium, and calcium in my food because they can interact adversely. And foods with too much tryptophan are at risk of actually killing me.

It all feels excessively complicated and maybe even a bit dangerous as I try to follow the thick packets of warnings and instructions, making charts and using timers to keep my foggy brain organized. But as anxious as I am to get the drugs and follow the instructions properly, I'm even more unnerved to require such rare medications. I'm appalled at what I'm putting into my body to fight a diagnosis we aren't even sure that I have. I tear up every time I see the lineup of pharmaceuticals and non-FDA-approved medications that litter my counter—now equally terrified of my failing health and treating it, too.

The medications have awful warning labels on them, and I take them in untested dosages and combinations. I take them off-label. They are normally prescribed for things like meningitis, cancer, tuberculosis, leprosy, and AIDS, and as I write this, I just took a radical one-dose treatment for malaria. It took me nearly eighteen hours to get up the courage to take that one—after reading online that it could kill my brain stem. And though I've told myself that won't happen, I hate that I stumbled upon the warning that it might.

It's terrible to be constantly on the lookout for potentially fatal reactions. To be sent home with strict instructions like: "If you can't get oxygen and you turn blue, go to the ER and ask for the antidote." And I hate that I keep getting oral thrush. But mostly, I'm terrified that one day I'll catch a superbug like *Clostridium difficile (C. diff)*. I'm fearful that, after all of this, it might be an inevitable outcome.

Hippocrates said food should be our medicine, and I believe in that, now more than ever. My body is run-down, beat up, and filled with pharmaceuticals, and when I think about what it is that *I* can control and how *I* can best support my body, I always come back to the power of nutrition.

I've done a lot of experimenting with my diet over the last decade. I've been paleo, keto, vegan, pescatarian—you name it. I've played around with calorie cycling, food combining, and intermittent fasting. I've always been chasing the right combination to feel at my best. And out of all the things I've tried, I found an anti-inflammatory diet to be the most impactful.

I've been gluten-free and dairy-free since 2012, and I rarely eat processed foods, refined sugars, or unhealthy oils. I can ensure this because nearly all of my meals are homemade; there were even a few years when I didn't eat in a single restaurant.

In 2018, I added even another layer to this, fine-tuning my nutrition even further when I began following an organic, whole-food plant-based diet. I'd never liked the idea of eating animals, anyway; I cried as a child any time my dad went hunting, and as an adult, I'd been trying to reduce my carbon footprint. So becoming plant-based, or vegan, was a lifestyle choice rooted in kindness and compassion that went way beyond my own health.

This is why, now here in 2020, I'm heartbroken that my new team of doctors has questioned this choice.

They say that Lyme can deplete someone's collagen, leading to further inflammation and pain. They've recommended instead that I follow a Lyme-specific autoimmune paleo diet. This is at least still anti-inflammatory and whole-food based, but it means I have to limit farmed grains and high-glycemic fruits, in addition to reintroducing animal protein.

I've wavered back and forth between believing the doctors on this or not—but ultimately, I've had to choose my own health. I need to get my life back. Figuring I've tried everything else already, I decided I might as well try this, too.

I've replaced my morning cup of coffee with organic, ceremonial-grade matcha tea. I make the exact same low-glycemic smoothie bowl every single day for breakfast, my recipe specifically created to fight inflammation and support both my failing thyroid and immune system. I stir in two scoops of collagen powder at the end, praying it will help my jaw joints heal. And I free-pour nut butter on top of it all to ensure sufficient caloric intake.

I eat it with a spoon, as the dentists have all told me that I can no longer use a straw, and I am pleased to report that it is quite delicious.

Lunches and suppers, however, are a bit more challenging.

I start by making a green smoothie, a celery juice, and a pureed vegetable soup. I focus on creating plant-centric meals, and then I force myself to eat some blended, organic, grass-fed beef or two ounces of canned, wild-caught salmon—both of which are soft enough for me to swallow without actually chewing. And as one would expect, I do find this to be quite awful.

My family has encouraged me to strive for progress and not perfection, yet I can't help but see danger and potential for failure everywhere I look. I insist on eating the exact same things every single week. I refuse to drink alcohol or eat any sugars, processed or natural, and I greatly limit my grains so as to not feed this hypothetical Lyme.

It's crucial I get this right. Exactly right.

My life is on the line.

This is the reason why, as strongly as I believe in my new Lyme diet, I am also choosing to believe in my restorative health practices. They will boost my immune system and open my drainage pathways to help detoxify the accumulation of toxicity, dying bacteria, and pharmaceutical burden. I've decided *this* will be the third and final angle of my treatment plan.

I've gone all in, spending thousands of dollars buying a far-infrared sauna, a hospital-grade air purifier, and a reverse osmosis water filtration system. I use only the cleanest, most natural options for both household and beauty products (even though I make sure to use very few of either). I even do my best to keep a clean mind, stay present, and surround myself with non-dramatic people. I take every chance I can to reduce toxicity in all areas of my life.

I also strive for routine and consistency in all things. I turn the lights out by nine each evening and get up every day at six (attempting nine hours of sleep, or at least forcing myself to keep the routine of lying there despite the insomnia). In the mornings, I sit peacefully by myself with my thoughts and my journal for at least an hour of emotional cleansing. I wear blue-light blocking glasses to not disturb my circadian rhythms. I take vitamins and supplements and drink half of my body weight in ounces of water every day. I use castor oil packs, have at least one detox bath with Epsom salts and baking soda every single day, and I attempt some form of movement (stretching, breathwork, or physical therapy exercises, whatever it is that my pained body can manage). And on Mondays, Wednesdays, and Fridays at two o'clock, I practice dry skin brushing, legs-up-the-wall pose, and sixty minutes in the far-infrared sauna. All of this followed by an icy-cold shower.

I'm motivated and energized to restore my health, and these practices give me a daily sense of purpose. Something to do and something positive to focus on. They give me a sense of control, and they give me a sense of hope.

I might have cried when I started eating animal protein again, thanking the fish as I gagged on my first bite, and again when I took my first dose of antibiotics. But it seems those things might be required, my penance to pay to get to the other side. So while I fear the dreaded Jarisch-Herxheimer reactions, also known as Herxing, I choose to see each pain as a reminder of the supposed infection they say I'm killing. Each pain a reminder that I'm taking control, sacrificing for a better and healthier life.

A war inside my body may have just begun, but I *am* persisting.

JJ

EIGHT YEARS OLD

Every morning before school, I waited until the last minute to see what my sister was wearing. Then I rushed into my room to try to copy her outfit exactly, or at least as closely as I could, from the items in my own closet.

I was lucky that our rooms were side by side and also that my mom had bought us a lot of the same things, as it only ever took a minute or two to transform myself into JJ's little twin.

"Ready!" I exclaimed as I proudly jumped out of my room with my arms outstretched. But upon seeing me, JJ just huffed and slammed her bedroom door. As a pre-teen, she was working on perfecting the attitude.

She always emerged calmly a few minutes later though, each time in a different yet equally great ensemble. And knowing I only had a few minutes to spare before the school bus arrived, I quickly took note of every detail of JJ's newest look and raced back into my room to change again. I riffled through my wardrobe for what I knew had to be there.

I stepped out proud of myself once more, in another nearly perfectly copied outfit.

"Ready again!"

We both wore our turquoise and pink striped spandex shorts, the ones with the white lace trim at the knee. Our mom had sewn us each a pair earlier that year, and they'd instantly become my favorite by far. We both had on white bobby socks and a baggy T-shirt, mine not exactly like hers, but close enough. And we each had a signature '90s headband in our hair—though mine was an ordinary sun-bleached blonde, and JJ's a more unique strawberry, we looked pretty close to twins, and I was proud of that.

"Mooooooom!" JJ yelled after taking one look at my nearly identical outfit.

I kept my head down and fiddled with the zipper on my backpack.

I did this every morning throughout third grade—I copied her outfit two or three times every single day, all the while feigning ignorance. I was committed; I was willing to change as many times as was necessary. The trick, however, was to time it correctly—so that the school bus arrived *before* JJ would have time to change again. Then there'd be no other choice than to go to school looking like twins.

I wasn't a morning person. I hated waking up early, hated walking to the bus stop, hated breakfast even (claiming nausea daily), but I did love that game. Copying JJ's outfit was my favorite part of every morning, and I liked to think she secretly enjoyed it too—the attention that I gave her and the fact that I adored her so much. So I pretended to be oblivious to her annoyance, and I kept the game alive, continuing to do it for the rest of the year.

JJ was the coolest. Only three years older than I was, yet mature beyond her years, I thought she knew everything. I was learning how to act, how to dress, and how the world worked just by watching her.

She could do no wrong in my eyes and seemed to excel at everything. She was the smartest in her class, and her success was becoming my motivation. I measured myself against her, holding myself to her standard. I never attempted to compete or outdo her because I knew that wasn't possible, I was just trying to keep up.

Even in dance, I was always trying to emulate JJ's movements. We were both training in ballet, tap, and jazz, and I tried to copy how she pointed her toes and elegantly placed her hands. I might have been cute, but I was clumsy—uncontrolled and awkward in my childish, overly flexible body. JJ had the poise of a real ballerina. When she got her first pair of pointe shoes, I followed her around the house for days, trying to balance all of my weight on just my bare, pointed toes.

She was pretty, fashionable, and creative, coming up with all of those really great outfits. And she was popular. I imagined she was probably the coolest person in our entire French immersion school, École St. Margaret. She even had a cool nickname, as her real name is Jennifer, yet throughout our entire lives, almost no one had ever called her that.

She was JJ.

Just JJ—like a rock star or a celebrity.

She drew attention everywhere we went, as strangers went out of their way to compliment her beautiful strawberry blonde hair—but I wasn't jealous of it. Rather, I was in awe. She was clearly the prettier, smarter one of us two, and everyone knew it and loved her for it. That was okay with me. I understood it because it was *I* who loved her the most out of all.

She was my big sister, and everything came naturally to her. She wasn't trying to be the best; she simply *was* the best, and I wanted to live up to that, too. I wanted to look and be exactly like my JJ, and copying her outfits had been my eight-year-old attempt at just that.

At that age, I copied JJ at every opportunity—with the exception of maybe just one.

Our parents had decided to build a new house that year. It would be modest in size, as most Canadian homes were. Tidy, with the warmth of a loving family home. And elegant, tastefully done according to my mother's refined aesthetic, in a palette of golden oak, dusty rose, and forest green. It was the spring of 1992, and our new home was set to be perfectly on trend with the latest style.

It was all going well. Our parents ran their own construction business; my dad led the day-to-day operations on site each day, while my mom handled the books, decorating, and landscaping. They were already a great team. I was confused when they sat JJ and me down one day, explaining that they wanted to include us in the excitement of this new build. They told us we could also be a part of the Johnson Construction team and have complete creative freedom in designing our own bedrooms.

I was shocked. Unsure what this would all entail, and unsure if our inclusion was a sensible decision.

In the weeks to come, however, I watched JJ make some really great choices. Inspired by Elizabeth of the *Sweet Valley Twins* series, she selected a mature color scheme of forest green and off-white that also happened to complement the rest of our new home. Yet even though I'd watched this, I didn't take as much into consideration as that. For the first time ever, I didn't follow JJ's lead.

I liked home design and had been rearranging my bedroom ever since I was old enough to walk. At every stage of childhood, I'd dragged, pushed, and pulled whatever pieces of furniture or home decor I was strong enough to move—learning with time to remove dresser drawers and walk the pieces inch by inch. I loved reimagining my space, organizing my toys, and displaying my stuffed animals just right. I was excited by the new opportunity I had been given. Exhilarated even. Commemorating that joy, I ended up selecting a bright salmon pink.

For everything. And my parents allowed it.

It read neon, a beautiful color perhaps to an eight-year-old, and not a terrible color for a single, individual item. The issue was that color adorned everything, everything that I had been allowed to choose: the walls, the curtains, the bedspread with its matching bed skirt. Even the wall-to-wall carpeting was pink. Bright salmon pink. As every single one of my selections came together in the end, the room created such a neon glow that it radiated down my mother's elegant hallway until it reached and ruined the kitchen.

It had to be fixed.

JJ's room, on the other hand, had turned out perfectly. Just like the rest of the house.

We only had to move three kilometers northeast. Our new house was located on an attractive suburban street, where other new and equally perfect homes had been popping up on the edge of the expanding town. It backed onto a large park with grassy green fields, the quintessential neighborhood rink, a playground, and a walking trail that encircled it all.

This was not only exciting to us kids, but it provided daily entertainment for the entire family as well. It was a place for us to play as much as a place for us to watch.

It was like having a big-screen television in our kitchen before the days of big-screen televisions. During family meals, we looked out the large windows and commentated on soccer games and flag football. We watched people walking their dogs and kids flying kites. But we also took to that park ourselves and learned to catch a baseball, as well as hit a golf ball. We skated on the hockey rink, played on the swings with Kyle and Kristin, and walked Tramp along the trail every single day—even if we did often lose her.

Beyond our park, there was nothing but wide open space. The edge of town. Vast prairie and a magnificent sky above an endless horizon. We found entertainment in that, too. With binoculars from my new bedroom window, I discovered I could watch the movies playing at the drive-in theatre outside of town, and if I tuned my radio just right, I could barely catch the audio, too. There was also the odd time during our first year living in that house when we watched a horse roam through the prairie and into our park, and we laughed, surprised to see a farm animal had entered the city. And that was the year the ostriches arrived.

I was an excitable kid—always walking on tiptoes, springing with every step. My heels never even came close to touching the ground. A happy and bouncy prancer I was. But that morning, I ran down the hallway toward the bedrooms, my little legs carrying me as fast as they could go. I burst into my parents' bedroom and jumped onto their bed, yelling at my dad to get up. Flustered and excited, I told him our entire backyard, the park, and the field beyond had all been filled with enormous birds.

"There are *ostriches* everywhere!" I exclaimed.

My dad startled awake at that, and an array of emotions washed across his still-groggy face—confusion predominantly, though also maybe some amusement. He allowed me to drag him by the hand as he crawled out of bed and padded sleepily down the hallway after me. He followed me like that all the way to the kitchen window, where I'd already gathered the rest of the family to look at the enormous flock of Canada geese that had landed in our backyard.

He laughed. They hadn't been ostriches, obviously, but I was thrilled with my discovery, nonetheless. The coffee was brewed, and the toast was made; it was the start of another great day. Our new house and that park were proving over and over a great combination of nature and city living. A perfect place for JJ and me to grow up together.

And together was how I liked it.

JJ and I entered every coloring contest held by the local *Times Herald*, each of us carefully perfecting our creations as we sat side by side at the kitchen table overlooking that park. We were both avid readers, and we frequented the Moose Jaw Public Library every two weeks together, each with a recycled Safeway bag in hand. We checked out the maximum number of books allowed, filling the flimsy plastic bags to the brim. Then we devoured the books once back at home. Sitting in our adjacent bedrooms overlooking that park, we read every single one, cover to cover.

JJ and I did everything together, and she'd been my best friend for as long as I could remember. I never understood why my classmates always complained about their siblings; JJ and I had never disagreed on anything—we'd certainly never fought. But some things *were* starting to change with us, I could feel that.

JJ had reached that pivotal age where kids seem to mature at an accelerated rate, going from child to teenager, ostensibly overnight. Our three-year age gap was starting to feel larger. I still enjoyed things like Barbies, whereas JJ had become more interested in sports. And for as much as we both loved that park, she now preferred to play catch with the football rather than race across my favorite monkey bars. We both had to try a little bit harder.

"I'll play Barbies with you for five minutes if you play football with me for ten," she proposed.

I paused, giving that some thought, glad to hear she was at least still proposing that we play together. "Why not Barbies for ten?"

"Well, seeing as you also like playing football, it's only fair that we would play it for longer," she explained matter-of-factly.

I had to give *that* some thought, too.

"Okay, Barbies for five and football for ten," I eventually agreed. Her explanation sounded logical enough, even though I recognized it wasn't exactly equal or fair. I followed along because that's what I always did, my big green eyes loyally watching her every move. I knew I would have been happy doing anything, just as long as we were together. My only objective was to spend time with her, have her attention, and be her friend.

I might have been eight, and she eleven, but I wasn't too young to understand that as long as we were together, I'd never be losing.

BATTLE

I thought I'd already endured the most severe pain possible.

It turns out I was wrong.

Immediately after the onset of my treatment at the end of May, my skin burned from the inside out. Bright red, angry streaks appeared on my hands and legs that were intensely sensitive to touch and temperature. Then those marks mysteriously rose up on my skin, prickly like sandpaper, and flaked off of my body in tiny sheets. And that subsequent moment of calm is what fooled me into a false sense of security.

The initial chaos of 2020 unfortunately continued as spring transitioned to summer, and the Lyme-guy's treatment made me worse—a lot worse. My list of twenty-five symptoms skyrocketed to thirty-seven.

I hadn't seen that coming.

Of course, I'd known that in order to treat some illnesses, a patient may need to get worse before they can get better; I knew chemotherapy could be like that. But what I didn't know, what I'd never fathomed, was that Lyme treatment was going to be similar.

I'm just along for the ride, it seems, as my protocol is changed, pulsed to stay one step ahead of a hypothetical bacterium. Each month, it allegedly unearths new areas of this so-called deeply rooted infection, and I Herx and I flare as a result.

It always starts with a paralyzing fatigue before I transition to nausea and double over from stomach pain. An eight-day, worse than usual, migraine usually follows. Then it's a thirty-six-hour attack of incapacitating electrocutions in my chest and days upon days of severe brain fog, crippling anxiety, and depression.

I'm in a constant state of agony now, with an unthinkable pain that has spread throughout most of my body. Weak, faint, and out of breath, I'm supposedly stuck in a state of backlogged toxic bacterial die-off. And my heart physically hurts.

It's a roller coaster of torture, continually ever-changing; I never know where the next dip and turn is going to take me. Impossible to predict that as summer faded into fall, I would struggle to walk. Or that the last time I tried to walk outside would end up being just that—the last time I tried.

It was a rare day, one where not only could I get out of bed, but I was willing to risk that ten minutes in the powerful sun would hurt my sensitive skin and eyes, and the sounds of neighborhood traffic and children would surely exacerbate my migraine.

I set out in a big floppy hat and long pants and sleeves, pulling the fabric down to protect even my fingers from the harsh rays of the sun. I held onto my husband's arm as we moved at what he jokingly referred to as my cripple speed. One shuffled foot, and then the next, we moved imperceptibly slowly, barely faster than standing still. Yet five minutes into our outing, I was already limping severely.

My right ankle was painfully arthritic and locking up on me, and my right calf felt like I had a permanent charley horse. My left kneecap and hip were on fire, and my right thigh was numb. My tailbone kept shooting electric pains that were taking my breath away, and my right oblique felt torn. Compensating for all of this, I had to shuffle stooped to one side with my hand pressing hard into my lower right quadrant—

but I could still appreciate that it was nice outside.

The sky was blue, the birds were singing, and big maple trees arched high overhead, their red leaves showing off the first signs of autumn. I whispered softly to a cottontail rabbit as I hobbled past it, a faint trace of a smile automatically attempted despite the screaming pain in my jaw.

And then I fell—as though shot through the leg, the pain blinded as it ripped through me. I dropped out from under my husband's grasp onto the street in an awkward and crumpled heap.

I'd never had one of my electrocutions in the leg before.

"I'm okay," I mumbled through my immobile jaw on instinct, those few painful words absolutely necessary as I saw the horrified look of concern on my husband's face. "Give me a second." I took a moment to gather myself, sitting there motionless in the middle of the road, catching my breath before I let him help me back up. I noticed that the cottontail rabbit was still watching.

"I can go get the car, Aim," he offered. "It's no problem. It'll only take a second for me to run and get it."

I shook my head slightly, not responding, not wanting to waste my jaw any further. I started my way back home. I stared at my feet and legs with a new intensity, slowly and methodically lifting and placing each foot one after the other. If I wanted to do this on my own, I knew I needed to stay focused.

"I don't mind," he continued. "I'd be back in no time. You could sit right here and wait."

Again I refused, this time by simply scrunching my nose slightly and shaking my head as I shuffled on. We hadn't even left our street yet; it would have been way too demoralizing to have to sit on my neighbor's lawn and await rescue. Even if walking was suddenly harder than I ever imagined.

My legs felt foreign to me, and my movements were jerky, robotic. My legs were no longer instinctually guiding me, and I was hyperaware of what it was taking to make each of them move. I had to focus intensely on the different muscle groups. One slow, awkward step at a time, my brain seemed unable to communicate the correct rhythm or order of events. Although even if I could get the rhythm right, I found I couldn't lift my feet high enough. I'd inadvertently angled my toes inward, knock-kneed and pigeon-toed, in an attempt to swing my feet out and forward instead of having to lift them. And every few steps, such a severe spasticity overtook my knee and hip joints that they refused to straighten or move at all. I shuffled and tripped and trembled until my legs buckled beneath me.

It was a bit like trying to run in a dream: a lot of effort to not get anywhere.

I had to stop after every house to try and catch my breath after that—regroup, and convince my legs to keep moving. They were worsening with every step. We were only three houses from home at that point, yet I was genuinely afraid I would not make it back.

"I can get the car," my husband said again.

This time, I outright ignored him. My entire focus was now dedicated to simply staying upright.

"Please, Aim, let me get the car."

Still, I continued. Progressively gripping his arm harder and leaning more heavily with each torturous step, so utterly fatigued, I could no longer respond. Instead, I dragged along my cement-filled shoes while fantasizing about mobility aids. A cane. A walker. A wheelchair. My legs popped and buckled with each attempted step, and my eyes filled with tears out of the sheer exhaustion, frustration, and embarrassment. Still, I refused to give up, no matter how many times my husband offered to get the car.

Until finally, he helped me into our house and back into my bed, where I have stayed ever since.

I've heard it's called ataxia, a loss of balance and coordination, and apparently encephalomyelitis could be the source of this loss of motor control—but I don't understand it. I get frustrated with myself, thinking that I'm not trying hard enough, though maybe the problem is that I'm trying *too* hard and thinking about it *too much*. However, it seems that no matter what I do, think or not think, cane or no cane, my legs simply don't work.

I'm bedridden at this point, relying on my husband for almost everything. He does all the cleaning, the cooking, and the errands. He helps me take my medications, microwave my dinner, and bathe. I feel absolutely worthless, only capable of stumbling and crawling to the bathroom as needed, in an oversized T-shirt and a pair of panties. The nerve pain prevents me from wearing anything else.

I can't socialize or even speak on the phone with my still-dislocated jaw—the pain there, too, only worsening. I can't even watch TV as the movements, sounds, and lights all make me nauseous. Nor can I read with my eyesight so blurry. And I try to avoid the internet because it just provokes anxiety.

I spend some of my days here, writing and researching a bit half-blindly on my phone, no longer able to make it to the laptop at my desk. But mostly, I pass the hours listening to audiobooks with my eyes closed. The pain prevents me from doing much of anything at all.

We joke that my tear ducts are the only thing on me that still work—which is both a sad statement and an accurate one. Sometimes I cry because I'm in pain, other times because I'm sad, but often my face leaks tears for no reason that I can understand at all. A result of some type of limbic seizure, maybe. Tears pour down my cheeks, yet even I have no idea why.

Between the unwashed hair and the constant state of dishabille, the collapsing, the crawling, the crying—it's not a good look. It's a pathetic existence, really. And none of the doctors are panning out. Unsure of any better options, I've had to continue treating with the Lyme-guy.

I despise going to the appointments each month. It's such an ordeal to get me all the way from my bed to the Lyme-guy's office—unable to walk, severely motion sick, the required mask triggering horrific facial pain, and the fear of contracting COVID with my single monthly outing.

But it might be *him*, above all, that I have come to despise the most.

I cry in the days leading up to the appointment and in the car with my husband on the way there. I even cry in the shoddy waiting room, knowing that I'll only have forty minutes with a dislocated jaw to accurately communicate to the guy the direness of my situation. I feel like my future is depending on me getting my words to him exactly right.

So as always, for this month's September appointment, I brought in notes. A typed, three-page monthly summary that my sister and husband helped me draft in advance. Yet even with those notes, due to my extreme brain fog, I still remained anxious about my ability to communicate with him, not confident at all in how much of my situation this Lyme-guy really understands. That is, with the exception of my very blunt opening statement—through my broken jaw *and* my mask, the words simply fell out. "I think you're killing me."

Yes, that time I was clear.

Still unfazed, the Lyme-guy reiterated what he'd been telling me all along. "You can take a break from the treatment at any time," he said.

But I knew I didn't want to do that—all I'd ever wanted was to hurry up and be done testing this theory of his.

"It's a marathon," he continued as if reading my mind. "Not a sprint. Most of my patients will require treatment for upward of a year, some even two. And we're only at what? Four months now? I'd like for you to stick with this. Give me six months, if you can, to really test it. Because it's around that six-month mark that we should start to see some changes. Some amelioration. Some sign of it working."

I stared at him, finding it hard to trust in his words when I knew I'd just spent the entire summer nosediving in the opposite direction.

"The more toxic and heavily infected a patient is to begin with, the worse the Herxing will be," the Lyme-guy went on as if he thought telling me that my infection was quite bad was somehow supposed to make me feel better.

He seemed to have an answer for everything, even for the questions I had yet to ask. Yet his answers never told me anything, nothing that helped anyway, so I didn't bother responding. Everyone in the room was already used to that.

"I'd say you have about an eighty percent chance of getting eighty percent better," he finished, interrupting my train of thought. And immediately, all of the air left my body.

An eighty percent improvement wouldn't give me my old life back. It wasn't good enough. His words, those percentages, swirled in my mind.

I only had an eighty percent chance of getting there?

An eighty percent chance of not-good-enough?

I couldn't breathe, yet I forced myself to move on in that moment—to find the tiniest sliver of bravery and stoicism deep inside of me. I knew I only needed enough to make it through the forty-minute appointment. I numbly handed him my notes.

I did not speak, whine or cry, faint, or throw up. And I certainly didn't waste any of our time discussing my emotions or fears. Instead, I sat silently and dug deep into the pot of muddled molasses that had become my brain, following along as the Lyme-guy read his printed copy of my notes aloud. Our same routine every time, every four weeks, the same.

I never admit to the Lyme-guy the constant monologue that plays in the back of my mind. How did I get here? Where did I go wrong? And I never admit that I'm struggling to accept when or where I would have even contracted Lyme disease, and that I still continually question if I even have it.

What is this, then?

What's wrong with me?

I have my family for support in that—my husband here, and my sister and parents up in Canada. I've always looked to them for explanations of the things in life I couldn't yet understand; like my dad's the type of person who questions everything, constantly curious and so constantly learning. I've always admired that quality in him. Even if sometimes that intellectual curiosity, the act of questioning, can sound a lot like distrust.

He's probably whom I get it from. Wondering every day if maybe the Lyme-guy is wrong, my doubts about this disease and the medical system as a whole are only compounded by the hesitation I hear in my dad's voice. And with every day that goes by, I wonder more and more about my dad's chronic back pain, wondering if it might be possible that we both have the same thing. Even if it has presented itself differently.

"Who is this guy you're seeing?" My dad asked over the phone after that appointment.

For my parents' sake, I tried to project a confidence that I didn't really have, a few forced sentences through a jaw that still refused to open. "He's a doctor," I mumbled. "He specializes in Lyme." Then, after an awkward silence, I added, "He went to one of the Ivy Leagues."

I knew it to be true—left alone waiting for him in his office one day, I'd studied quite closely the framed degrees hanging on his wall. And I've certainly done my research since. Day after day on my phone, I've gotten a little creepy; it's amazing how far back into someone's life you can get with enough hours and the internet at your disposal. But even though the Lyme-guy seems legit (strange Halloween pictures on Facebook aside), I still have my doubts. And I can hear in my dad's voice that he does, too.

I don't know what to say to comfort my parents. My decline feels counterintuitive and counterproductive. It doesn't feel right.

Nothing in me feels right.

I'm afraid the Lyme-guy's treatment might be killing more of me at this point than the hypothetical infections. My husband and I agonize about the impact this is having on my body—never sure at which point we should be rushing back into Urgent Care or Emergency, when I am now *perpetually* in a state of emergency.

Yet we recognize those trips in the past have never proved fruitful. Neither the Lyme-guy nor any other doctor has ever been able to explain my pain. What exactly is happening inside of my body or jaw. How dangerous or life-threatening the electrocutions may be. Why they keep happening. Or, maybe most importantly, how to stop them. Doctors' offices, specialists, and ERs alike have been at a loss all this time.

So with no explanations and no more tests to run, I stay put and continue to suffer at home, clinging to the hope that the Lyme-guy actually knows what he's talking about. My research tells me that a Herx reaction should only occur when medications are killing off an infection, so if I am indeed Herxing, this would not only be a confirmation of a Lyme diagnosis but a sign that the treatment for it is working.

The obvious question is: Am I actually Herxing?

For right or for wrong, with no answers, we cross our fingers, and we continue to handle it alone—without any family within a thousand miles and not wanting to lean on the few new friends we've just met here. Besides, we're still pretty isolated due to the global pandemic. The Canadian border is sure to remain closed for the foreseeable future, what with one million recorded deaths and the number of confirmed cases worldwide hitting thirty million just recently at the beginning of September.

The UN now warns of a potential mental health crisis due to this forced isolation, fear, and uncertainty, and that's *definitely* something I can relate to.

I feel trapped here, desperate to escape not only this house, but free myself from the prison that is my body. I live alone in my head, day after day, with only my confused thoughts, questions, tormented emotions, and pain to keep me company. I'm afraid I'll never live pain-free again.

And unable to speak, I just constantly cry.

WASKESIU

TEN YEARS OLD

Loaded up in the family van, ready to head out on summer holiday, I found myself still humming the tune from weeks prior. I'd been timid during the end-of-school performance of that fifth-grade musical, *Family Vacation*—hiding in the background while on stage, with zero concept of notes, pitch, or key. But secretly, I dreamed that I could have sung the solo.

It may have been obvious to everyone around me that my talents lay more on the athletic side of things, but at ten, I wasn't sure where I fit in the world. I was shy and quiet, and my teachers often expressed surprise whenever I spoke up in class. Out in public, my parents were always asking me to speak louder and clearer. My voice was rarely above a whispered mumble.

At home it was different. I felt comfortable to express myself in all things creative. I liked arts and crafts, sewing, choreography, and dance, I even liked to write my own songs and record myself singing them. So there, in the comfort of the family van at the onset of our vacation, I didn't hesitate to sing loud and clear. We were waiting anyway, with Dad still inside the house, refilling his coffee cup again before we could depart.

"Traveling down the road, hauling quite a load. Seeing things we've never seen before…"

Our family often went on vacation, exploring both Canada and the United States. We saw the majestic Canadian Rockies and the ever-so-tacky-and-sparkly Las Vegas. We went to Disneyland (the happiest place on earth) and saw the carvings at Mount Rushmore. We never flew, rather we drove everywhere in the family van—motion sick and loaded up on antiemetics perhaps, but even that couldn't take away my joy. And every summer, my parents made time for a trip up to Waskesiu. It was our constant. And to me, it was a magical place.

Located in northern Saskatchewan, the Prince Albert National Park was only a five-hour drive from Moose Jaw, yet in those five hours, we were transported into another world. Gone were the expansive wheat fields and prairie pastures. This was the raw wilderness of the northern boreal forest: towering white birch and evergreens that went on endlessly, and massive, pristine lakes with rocky shores.

The little town of Waskesiu stood at the center of it all, the only hamlet in the entire park. It was adorably minuscule, dwarfed by the breadth of the surrounding wilderness—a thousand nearby hiking trails yet only a handful of streets, a general store, a few bits of clothing and souvenirs, and ice-cream shops galore. As many flavors as you could imagine.

My favorite part, was that the forest and the town alike brimmed with animals. The roll of film in our family camera quickly filled with slightly out-of-focus images of elk wandering through town and me happily sitting on the ground feeding the squirrels and ducks. One time, while walking along the path that paralleled the shoreline, a massive dragonfly even landed on JJ's small shoulder, amazing us all.

It was much larger than any dragonfly we'd ever seen before, otherworldly and ethereal in its beauty. Its translucent wings and iridescent body scintillated in the sun in a multitude of colors—it fascinated me. But always-cool, of course, JJ continued walking on.

I wasn't surprised by that.

The unexpected part was that the oversized dragonfly appeared equally unfazed and stayed on JJ's shoulder, riding along for an hour while we continued our walk around town. Even as we went in and out of the shops. I was in awe of the mystical fairy-like creature, our proximity to something so wild and free that somehow seemed completely comfortable with our presence. Though I was a bit jealous it had chosen to ride on JJ's shoulder and not mine, the encounter solidified in my mind that my sister was uniquely special and that every part of Waskesiu was extraordinary. It was the stuff storybooks were made of.

It wasn't only me who was drawn to it. Waskesiu was a popular travel destination, one that never felt crowded thanks to the expanse of the wilderness, but accommodations did sell out quickly each season. And my dad wasn't exactly one to plan ahead.

Dad blamed the difficulty of coordinating time away with projects at work, yet I suspected he simply preferred spontaneity as our trips were always booked last minute. As a result, we stayed at a different place every year.

The cabins were by far my favorite. I loved waking up each morning and venturing straight outside, where the dew was fresh on the trees, and the damp smell of the pine forest filled my lungs. I knew, before I even stepped off the little porch, that the earth would feel spongy with pine needles under my feet. And the towering pines above would dapple the morning sun in such a way that, when I tilted my face upward to listen to the songbirds, ripples of sunlight would dance across my face.

I liked to leave nuts and seeds on the railing so that I could watch the squirrels through the small cabin window later in the day. Amazed by their tiny little hands stuffing so many treasures into their already-bulging cheeks. There were characters to see, pinecones to pick, and the thrill of a potential bear sighting when we stayed in one of the cabins.

At the hotel, however, I felt fancy. I was forever on my best behavior at the Hawood—though I only ever pronounced it the "Haaaaa-wood," trying to act older than my age and faking a pretentiousness I'd only ever seen in the movies.

It was classy, especially their dining room. It served high-end dishes like New York steak, Lac La Ronge pickerel, and exotic side dishes I'd never even heard of—things like risotto. I always made sure to blend in like I belonged there. Except, of course, for the time I screamed when a bug suddenly emerged from my salad and then scampered across my plate. I'd been telling my mom for years that vegetables were gross, and *this* had finally proved my point.

But bugs in the salad or not, we ate at the Hawood every summer, followed by a family stroll down to one of the local ice cream shops. I discovered pralines and cream, Mom favored mint chocolate chip, JJ chose maple, and reliable 'ol Dad refused to try anything except plain 'ol chocolate.

We rented funny bikes in town, too, tandem ones and quadricycles (the kind where entire families rode together). We rented canoes and kayaks and hiked the many trails exploring the wilderness—the forest and the untamed beaches. And we always brought our boat with us to Waskesiu because the lakes up north were massive.

Spanning so far we couldn't even see the opposing shoreline, it was like we were conquering the ocean whenever we set off in search of adventure. Yet somehow, my dad always managed to find us a tiny little island with a remote beach, completely undiscovered and untraveled by anyone before us. He would run our boat up onto its shore.

Mom and JJ would immediately head off in search of treasures. JJ had an affinity for rock collecting, and Mom liked to bring back pieces of driftwood for her garden at home—neither of which I really understood—but I didn't pay them much attention. Dad and I had our own adventures ahead of us.

We'd proudly throw on our matching Cons and set off to explore the rugged little piece of land, looking for signs of wildlife. All the while, Dad would regale me with stories that may or may not have been entirely true, but I listened with wide eyes anyway. I was captivated and enthralled by his knowledge, his storytelling, his imitation of an elk bugle, and the excitement of exploring the wild terrain together.

We'd only reconvene with Mom and JJ once our explorations and collections were complete. Dad would build us a fire and carve branches into long sticks while Mom unpacked the hotdogs and marshmallows from the cooler for a campfire lunch.

The main event would soon follow when it was warm enough for us to go tubing: JJ and I lying side by side on our bellies, gripping the handles of the inflated donut, talking and laughing as we bounced and skidded across the water.

We often spent time on the smaller and less popular Hanging Heart Lakes for that. These were a series of mid-sized lakes connected to one another by shallow marshy channels. Peaceful passages narrowly cut through the forest, the very center no more than three feet deep—barely deep enough for a boat like ours to pass. But taking these hidden waterways was the only way to access some of these lakes. In doing so, we could often find an entire lake on which to spend the whole day, with much calmer waters for tubing. It would often just be us out there, alone with the echoing calls from loons all around.

On such a day, JJ and I opted to stay on the tube while we traveled through one of those channels. Dad slowed the boat to a troll as he approached the posted speed limit, and JJ and I shifted our weight backward automatically to ensure we wouldn't tip over. We settled in for the brief commute. Lying lackadaisically on the neon pink and lime green tube, with the warm sun shining down on us, we succumbed to the tranquil intermission in our tubing excitement. I let my mind wander to the little creatures who might live in this marshy world.

Tree stumps stuck out of the water along the shoreline, framing our path, and as we traveled up the narrows, I leaned down close—allowing my face to hover only inches above the crystal clear waters. The sun glinted, illuminating the world below, and I dangled my fingers, barely brushing the surface. I scouted for minnows and watched the reeds and the lily pads, with their pretty pink flowers that tickled our trailing toes as we passed. I imagined there would be tiny little green frogs, big ugly toads, and those funny little bugs that zipped and weaved across the surface of still water.

I watched for it all.

When suddenly, up ahead of us on the boat, we saw our mom jump out of her seat. She appeared to be speaking frantically to Dad about something, though with our tube floating fifty feet behind the boat and the quiet hum of the motor between us, I couldn't hear what was going on.

The two of them started waving excitedly to us and pointed out in the distance, where I finally saw the reason for the commotion. There, emerging from the forest up ahead, only fifteen feet away from the boat, was an enormous bull moose. At over six feet tall and well over a thousand pounds, it was a thrilling sight for sure. But as the moose started to move slowly in our direction, my mom's look of excitement quickly changed to one of alarm. And JJ and I, lying beside each other on the tube, automatically stilled.

Through the trees, through the marshy tree stumps, the moose walked straight into our channel.

I stared transfixed at the scene before me—my focus flicking between the moose and my parents on the boat up ahead, now clearly arguing. We couldn't hear what they were saying, but Mom was apparently insisting that Dad speed up; he had to get us out of there. Her only two children were out in the water, exposed and alone. Yet Dad was uneasy, certain that he had no other choice but to stay the course due to the shallow waters. The motor couldn't be lowered any further. We only had this one speed.

"Girls. Don't. Move." We heard our dad yell out. The moose was now fully in the water, a dark, ominous form plodding toward us.

Possible outcomes flooded our dad's mind. He could see the moose was on a direct path to collide with our thin nylon rope, the only lifeline connecting his kids to the boat. And it would be disastrous if the rope got accidentally entangled with a moose—especially a panicking one—one end of the rope tied to the boat, and the other end tied to his children. A wild bull moose certainly did not belong in the middle of all that.

Dad couldn't speed up.

But he was afraid to stop.

So, without any other option, our dad calmly drove on. The boat and our tube inched up the channel, and my mind flitted to the irony that our family loved moose. In fact, every night after dinner in Waskesiu, we drove through the National Park intentionally trying to find them. Squinting into the darkness through the blur of evergreens, we were always trying to catch a glimpse of a bear or an elusive moose in a swamp.

Based on the look on our mom's face, I was guessing *this* was becoming too near for comfort.

The moose was closing in.

While on the tube, JJ and I had not moved. We were frozen, still, and silent. We did not speak to one another. We did not even flinch. We simply stared wide-eyed at the moose. His massive chest parted the way through the reeds and the lily pads, and I couldn't tell if he was walking or swimming. My young mind was unable to fathom that this animal could be so impossibly tall to walk straight across our channel.

Finally, the moment came. Our paths converged.

We lay helpless on the tiny floating tube—JJ on my right side and the moose now directly beside me on the left. The moose's head was bigger than even the tube we lay on. And he looked at us with his big, black, cartoonish eyes, and our wide eyes stared right back at him. We were so close I could have reached out and petted him, touched his comical, big, bulbous nose. There was a part of me that even wanted to, though some instinct in the back of my mind kept me frozen in place.

Time seemed to stop with our stare-down.

Then, at what seemed a snail's pace, we floated past. The tube continued forward, while the moose, perhaps a bit curious, seemed somehow untroubled by our presence. He *waited*, politely allowing us to cross first. He only went on his way once we were clear. And our heads swiveled around to the other side to watch him cross behind us, barely missing our little toes.

We stared as we left him behind. My dad followed up the length of the channel toward the safety of open water again, while the moose finished crossing, emerged from the water on the opposing shore, and disappeared into the trees once more. The moment was gone, but the memory of our face-to-face encounter would be frozen in each of our minds forever.

Waskesiu really was magical.

COMPLICATED

I'm sick—really sick—and I don't know if I should be blaming the pandemic or the medical system as a whole, but I feel like I'm all on my own here trying to solve it. Trying to understand. And trying to understand Lyme disease is proving to be a near-impossible task.

Lyme is complicated. It is difficult to test and to treat. However, it is also greatly misunderstood and often goes completely unrecognized. The "facts" are inconsistent and constantly changing: within the medical community, within public perception, and especially on the internet. Yet the worst parts are the politics and debate surrounding it. The issue begins simply in an attempt to define it, and even to name it. The controversy over a chronic form of Lyme disease stems from the question of its mere existence.

I hadn't previously known that it was so controversial, and I quickly became afraid of being duped. I was afraid this was all a scam—that these alternative doctors were charlatans out to steal my money. I'm still not entirely convinced that they aren't. It's pretty hard to believe the Lyme-guy's theory of chronic Lyme disease when I'm not sure Lyme disease is even real. It's unfathomable to me that the medical community can be so divided on a subject.

For my own sanity, I know I need to understand it better. My research tells me that while issues can be found in many agencies—the government, CDC, FDA, Big Pharma, state medical licensing boards, and the health insurance industry—at the root are the Lyme disease guidelines put forth by the IDSA (Infectious Diseases Society of America).

I've learned that Lyme is a multi-faceted infectious disease. It is caused by bacteria that have been around for millions of years, but the disease itself is far from being fully understood. It only first became reportable thirty-four years ago, and sufficient research studies haven't been conducted yet to consider the complexity of the individual nuances or the many infections that Lyme patients might face. Yet the IDSA guidelines continue to be based on this lack of research and, therefore, remain insufficient as well.

This has resulted in a very conflicted medical community filled with skeptics, conspiracy theorists, and old-school doctors who do not even believe that Lyme disease can exist in a chronic form beyond the first twenty-eight days. They acknowledge that the patient is ill, but they have no concrete explanation for it.

These old-school doctors only see Lyme as an immediate reaction to a bite from an infected deer tick carrying the bacteria *Borrelia burgdorferi*—a microscopic little bug called a spirochete, a corkscrew-shaped worm. They consider the infection "easy to cure, no matter how advanced the case" and follow the standard IDSA guidelines for antibiotic therapy, which can range from ten to twenty-eight days. And if caught early enough, this treatment can be successful, because in its first acute stage, the Lyme infection is early localized and has not yet spread throughout the rest of the body.

The issue is that few people do catch it right away. People often don't see the tick that bit them nor develop an erythema migrans rash, so they don't know to immediately start antibiotics. And with time, as the infection goes undiagnosed and untreated, the bacteria will multiply and spread all throughout the body. The spirochetes infiltrate tissues and take up residence, especially preferring the collagen and myelin-rich areas of the body, until the infection eventually progresses into a very dangerous condition called late-stage Lyme disease. This is what the Lyme-guy thinks must have happened to me.

Supposedly, infections can lay dormant for years. Similar to other diseases like cancer, the spirochetes will go into a stealth mode, morphing into persister cells and adopting various shapes and sizes. They can create microcolonies, secrete biotoxins, and even build a protective biofilm around themselves, making it nearly impossible for the immune system to find them and fight.

It is estimated that this occurs in five to fifteen percent (though some have estimated as high as thirty-five percent) of the nearly half a million cases of Lyme disease each year in the United States. This means two million people could be suffering from chronic symptoms of Lyme disease by the end of 2020. Yet while the medical community is wasting precious time debating whether the persisting symptoms are being caused by an active infection, a triggered autoimmune reaction, or some combination of both, old-school doctors are simply giving up—condemning their patients to live with chronic and debilitating symptoms. As with the timeframe for a quick and easy treatment long passed, the disease only gets harder to treat and impossible to cure. And the IDSA guidelines are completely useless by that point.

What these patients will now need is a prolonged treatment that goes against those outdated IDSA guidelines, but many have deemed that approach too dangerous.

It is a path of great ambiguity, with no real governance and no test to determine if the infection is ever completely destroyed. The goal instead for these patients is simply to kill enough of the infection so that the immune system regains control, the body finds homeostasis, and the patient achieves some type of remission. Though often, future relapses will occur, and further treatments may still be required.

Adding to this complexity, the guidelines don't even take into account that Lyme disease is a lot more than a single infection of *Borrelia burgdorferi*. Ticks can transmit multiple infections in a single bite, and these co-infections are often worse than the *Borrelia* itself—not only tougher to diagnose but tougher to treat, too. And when someone's immune system becomes so compromised like that, patients end up acquiring opportunistic secondary infections and associated disorders as well.

In fact, the Lyme-guy doesn't even use the term "Lyme" to refer to what he thinks he's treating me for, and I've found myself constantly wondering what it is exactly he thinks that I have. Chronic Lyme, neurological Lyme, late disseminated Lyme, late-stage Lyme, late persistent Lyme? Even with all that, I still hear old-school doctors in the community continue to use the term "post-treatment Lyme disease syndrome"—though that seems like a different thing altogether, in my opinion.

I guess I'm learning that "Lyme," whichever version of the name might you use, may not even be the right term at all. The more accurate term, encompassing all of a person's co-infections, would be tick-borne illness or tick-borne disease. But either way, regardless of what name you might hear or choose to use, it's important to understand that Lyme is often more than a single infection. More than a single illness.

Further, there are a great variety of ways in which those illnesses might present. The variety is so great, in fact, that some people exposed to the infections feel it immediately, whereas others may remain asymptomatic indefinitely, and the rest fall somewhere in between. Some may develop only a handful of mild symptoms, but for others, the disease can become completely incapacitating. The disease can even be fatal.

How one reacts to Lyme comes down to the exact mix of the patient's individual infections, their preexisting health and genetics, immune system, and even their environment. And it seems that neither the guidelines nor our medical system were designed for something as complicated as that.

Our medical system was designed with our general family doctor as our first line of defense. But I've found it's not uncommon for them to tell you, "Only one concern can be addressed at today's appointment." I've even had family doctors stand in the doorway with their hand still resting on the doorknob—they never even fully entered the room for my appointment, let alone closed the door. A clear indication that my time allotment wouldn't be very long.

Rarely do we encounter someone who takes the time to look at the body as a whole or try to get to the root of what is causing our symptoms. Our medical system, unfortunately, is one designed to manage illness rather than restore wellness. It is a system in which doctors are so over-scheduled that they don't have time to listen to a patient with ten symptoms, or twenty, and certainly not thirty or forty. Especially not fifty-six. Although even if a doctor did listen, most are not sufficiently educated on tick-borne illness, which only further exacerbates misconceptions.

Most old-school doctors following the guidelines don't even think to test for Lyme, falsely believing that it's rarer than it actually is. Many still operate under the assumption that Lyme only exists on the East Coast and must always present with a bullseye rash—but neither statement is true. Insects don't abide by state lines (nor do the migratory birds on which they attach), so Lyme disease doesn't either. And less than thirty percent of patients will ever develop the "telltale" rash.

Of course, even if your family doctor did think to test you, I've learned that testing for Lyme through the current American standard screening is only about fifty percent accurate, mostly only catching the acute cases. And this only compounds the misbelief that Lyme is rare and that the infection can only be active in those first twenty-eight days.

The Lyme community suggests you need to follow an alternative route, see a Lyme-literate medical doctor (LLMD)—like apparently my Lyme-guy is—and get tested at a specialty lab. But then, because none of this is mainstream, I've also learned that everyone around you is going to question it. Only adding to the doubts and the fears in your head. And you'll have to pay out of pocket for all of it, as insurance companies refuse to cover anything beyond what is stated in those outdated IDSA guidelines.

I'm currently paying thousands of dollars each month for my treatments; my insurance claims and health spending account charges get denied weekly. Yet I remind myself that at least I'm receiving a treatment—getting a chance to see if what I have really could be Lyme. As one of the most difficult challenges that patients face is that most doctors aren't even willing to take the risk of talking about the possibility of Lyme, let alone treat it. In the past, medical licenses have been suspended and even revoked for treating a patient against those outdated IDSA guidelines. So still to this day, many doctors avoid any association with Lyme disease, and the patients are avoided, too—disregarded in our medical system, pushed aside, considered too complicated to help, and not worth the time or risk.

It's a broken system and one that extends even further than I could have imagined.

Growing up in Canada, I'd always heard there was a miraculous place where you could go in the States. It was a place where an entire team of brilliant doctors would be assembled just for you, and teams of specialists from all different domains would work together to solve your mystery and save your life. It sounded a lot like the TV show *House*.

All you had to do was show up.

I'd been saving the Mayo Clinic as my last resort, my plan B, my Hail Mary pass. Holding on to the hope that if my shotgun approach—the different doctors, these treatments, this Lyme-guy's theory—didn't work out, I'd simply go there. And with how I've been declining lately, my breaking point came after this month's November appointment.

I'd given the Lyme-guy the six months he'd asked for, yet all I'd done was decline that entire time. I was frustrated, distrustful, and still not convinced that what I had was even Lyme. I was pretty confident that the Lyme-guy was guessing—an educated and experienced guess, sure, but guessing nonetheless. At every appointment, he told me something slightly different, and I'd spend the next four weeks clinging to those words. Rereading our notes of the exact verbiage he'd used, I'd try to buy in and believe what he had said, have faith in the current month's treatment. But without fail, he'd always contradict himself at the next appointment, and the constant switching of theories and medications was leading me to believe that he didn't know what he was doing.

His theory that Lyme was trapped in my body, trapped in my dislocated jaw and preventing it from healing, was starting to feel unsound.

I was hoping to leave him for something better—a diagnosis I could have confidence in and a treatment that might actually work. But between the COVID restrictions and my being too sick to travel, I didn't get to go anywhere. We had to speak with the Mayo Clinic via telemedicine. It wasn't ideal, not at all how I'd always imagined it.

Here at my desk, as always in my ratty sweatpants and hoodie, my husband joined me for a series of calls. I tried to sit still as he spoke for me—explaining to the Mayo Clinic my symptoms, the theory of Lyme disease, and the paths I'd already tried. We hadn't packed our suitcases yet, but we *were* ready to go. My husband and I had already calculated and discussed how, with COVID and my pain, we would have to drive the thousand miles out there rather than fly. However, hour after hour, we were passed around the Mayo Clinic from person to person (everyone claiming "not their department"). They didn't even sound that interested in helping me, when they could clearly see my plight.

I couldn't speak, I couldn't walk. We were confused that they hadn't immediately admitted me as a new patient. This was proving harder and more time-consuming than either of us had expected.

Time passed, and my excitement and my hope were starting to morph into trepidation. My husband paced back and forth in our small room, no longer able to sit still in front of the screen. I wished I could do the same. My heart rate and breath were a bit irregular, while back and forth, back and forth across the room he went. All I could do was wring out my hands, twist and stretch in my seat, and try to ignore the slight tremor building in my arms.

I had no voice of my own, yet my entire life was riding on the success of these calls.

The entire day passed like that. Each time we were transferred to a different department head for consideration (including the infectious disease department because Lyme *is* considered to be an infectious disease), we had to repeat our story all over again. Our hope rose with each telling, but it immediately fell again with each transfer. It was beyond exhausting, listening to the same conversation over and over, my trauma minimized with each rendition. And though our hope did rise, it rose a little less and fell a little harder each time.

My pain was escalating out of control. My tears were threatening. We waited on pins and needles for the final call to come through, both of us trying to keep our last sliver of hope alive.

"Your case will now go before the board," a lady told us. "Thank you for your interest in the Mayo Clinic." But I thought her voice sounded a bit too formal to be good news, as it completely lacked any compassion or personality. "We'll be contacting you in one to three business days with the final decision," she finished as she abruptly hung up. The tone behind her words rang out loud and clear—this wasn't going to be good. My husband and I just stared at each other as the words "one to three business days" echoed in our minds.

They emailed me the denial within the hour.

I wasn't sure they'd even considered me.

The Mayo Clinic, we'd come to find out, is old-school. They do not deal with, or maybe even believe in, late-stage or chronic Lyme disease.

I wanted to scream at them that I wasn't sure I believed in it either—yet I still needed help. That's *why* I'd come to them. But I understand now that it wouldn't have changed a thing.

I'd read previously that Lyme patients get marginalized, overlooked, and ignored. Cast out and neglected. I'd read that the medical uncertainties and controversies surrounding Lyme have resulted in many doctors choosing to avoid these complicated patients and tick-borne illnesses altogether. I'd read that having Lyme is like having cancer, but without the structured support of the medical community. I just hadn't realized the accuracy of any of those statements until this week.

Not until it was *I* who was marginalized—for even suggesting that I might have it.

My eyes have been opened now. And I know there are so many others out there, like me, who desperately need help. Lyme disease is a growing epidemic, the fastest-growing vector-borne disease in the United States, in fact, yet advancement has remained a struggle. "Public awareness might be at an all-time high right now, but concern from the medical community is at an all-time low."[1]

This experience has left me even more afraid, with no backup plan and no other choice but to navigate this controversial and informational minefield all on my own, finding my way outside of the mainstream medical system. Though I suppose "mainstream" did only ever fail me, anyway. It never hesitated to provide me with an entire bottle of narcotics for only $4.37 or a bottle of tranquilizers for $1.96, but accurate testing to determine what was actually wrong with me was never offered at all. Nor were any suggestions on how I might attempt to resolve it.

So here I am, resigned to continue on the Lyme-guy's alternative path—very much still struggling to trust and very much still continuing to decline. I feel trapped in that his clinic is the only one I've found even willing to take me. And I struggle to accept his treatments when I know opinions differ greatly on the appropriateness and risk. But above all, I'm still struggling to believe a diagnosis as I attempt to find my way in a world that only vaguely believes in Lyme.

Marginalized, isolated, and alone.

This is completely unacceptable.

AJ

ELEVEN YEARS OLD

It was during my 1994 dance festival performance when two girls carried me in the splits—one foot balancing precariously on each of their shoulders as they walked dramatically onstage. I floated high in the air above the other dancers, and all eyes were on me.

I wasn't sure I liked the feeling.

I'd always thought I was too tall and had been uncomfortable with any form of attention, but I was chosen for the role because I was stick-thin and light and the most flexible one at my dance school. I'd even been nicknamed Gumby after the excessively bendy green toy.

That ability of mine was both a gift and a disadvantage. It took a lot of strength for me to accomplish that pose—to not allow my torso to drop too far into my natural over-split, as that would have dangerously compromised the stability of the hold. But I managed it. The performance was a success, and the crowd cheered. I felt both a little uncertain and proud afterward in the crowded lobby of the auditorium, where my parents and Grandma Smolinski congratulated me.

Despite another successfully completed performance, I was questioning if my time as a dancer was coming to an end. For nearly ten years, I'd enjoyed the actual dancing part, but I no longer felt that I fit in with the other girls.

At only eleven, I'd been placed in a group with much older dancers, many of them already old enough to drive. I frequently found myself sitting alone in the changing room while they chatted animatedly before class. I tried not to draw any attention to myself, tried not to take up any space at all. Keeping my eyes down and slouching my already too-tall frame, every day I just tried to disappear. I even went so far as to tune out their conversations so they wouldn't think that I was eavesdropping. I knew how much teenagers hated when kids did that.

It wasn't much better for me in the studio either. Both the dance environment and the act of dancing itself were starting to stifle me. I needed more.

It didn't bother me that I'd developed what my parents considered to be a significant case of asthma. I coughed incessantly anytime I ran, as well as all throughout the night—a dry, hacking cough that kept the whole house awake, and forced me to sleep sitting straight up. To me, it wasn't much different from the nosebleeds I'd suffered in first grade. At upward of three times a day, I hadn't found them especially noteworthy; rather, they were simply a part of my normal life. Like falling off the playground and scraping a knee. Unfortunate, sure, maybe even a story to tell in the schoolyard—but nothing more.

Besides, my mom never gave me any reason to worry; she always tried to carry those types of things on our behalf. She sat with me while I coughed, just as she'd sat with me while I'd bled—always the picture of patience and calm, even if secretly wondering to herself when this was ever going to stop. Wondering at what point she should be taking me to the hospital. Wondering, always wondering, and praying she was doing everything right.

Dr. James eased her mind on this. He was soft-spoken to the point of mumbling, reserved to the consequence of being socially awkward, and always extremely kind. He was the type of small-town doctor whose door was always open, whether you had an appointment or not. He answered his own phones and was even willing to make house calls. And Dr. James had found my nosebleeds to be "quite normal," attributing the onset to an allergy from all the construction dust at school, while for the asthma, he provided medications, inhalers, and referrals to specialists.

It all improved with time—I was well cared for, both by him and by the conscientiousness of our parents. And I had no intention of letting any of it get in my way.

I was excited to play football, volleyball, and basketball on the school teams at École St. Margaret, in addition to fastball in the city league where my dad volunteered as a coach. I'd been discovering that not only was I naturally athletic with my tall and slim build, but I also enjoyed being competitive. So I tolerated the coughing and my weekly respiratory therapy appointments at the hospital—my focus remained entirely on sports.

I was falling in love with basketball.

I'd watched every one of JJ's high school games that season and been enamored, drawn to the fast pace and excitement. And I attributed a lot of her team's growth and success to the man at the center of it all. An import from a big American city, Coach A was special. I could tell that right away.

It wasn't long before he became a friend of our entire family, and I got to know him personally as well. He did everything in a hurry, yet always managed to come across as laid-back. He was a bit older than my parents, but not overly concerned with rules or following what others might expect of him. He was funny, and maybe even a little weird—but in a good way, in the way that only some of the best people are. Unafraid of being himself, Coach was always making jokes and playing pranks. He constantly teased my mom, knowing he could get a rise out of her. On more than one occasion, he jumped out of a random hiding place dressed as a gorilla, scaring the living daylights out of me. And without possibly knowing the impact it would have, Coach A gave me my very own nickname.

He approached me in the Peacock Collegiate gym, where I'd been shooting hoops with some other kids down on the court during the halftime break of JJ's game.

"Hey AJ," Coach called casually in my direction. "You wanna play the next half?"

I stared at him blankly, the basketball in my hands forgotten. I looked behind me. I turned back to him. Coach A was always joking around, but I didn't understand where he was going with this one.

I stood there motionless, unsure what to say, when he abruptly turned and walked away from me—apparently not bothering to wait for my response. He grabbed an extra jersey from a bag behind the bench and threw it at me. The clump of fabric hit me square in the chest; my arms, like my mind, were too slow to react. Then, without missing a beat, Coach proceeded to walk over to the scorekeeper's table and scribble something on the official roster.

It took me a second, maybe two, before I followed him over there. I didn't feel it was really my place, but I knew I needed to see it for myself. And there, on the last line of the official roster, was a name. The first time I'd ever seen it written.

No first name, no last name—AJ.

Just AJ—followed by the number thirteen.

With trembling fingers, I looked down and unfolded the jersey in my hands. In the boldest of red was the number thirteen. He hadn't been joking.

I'd never worn a real basketball jersey before, and I slipped the foreign garment over my T-shirt in a stunned silence. Then I hurried over to the empty bench and sat awkwardly on the farthest end. Not wanting to infringe on any of the space for the real players, I imagined when they returned, they would all be judging my sudden presence—wondering why a kid was wearing their team jersey. Wondering why a kid was even there.

The court looked huge from this new vantage point, and I sat meekly, nervous and shy, trying not to fidget or show my intimidation. The rest of the girls soon joined me, and the second half of the game continued. I cheered cautiously alongside them, doing my best to try to blend in. But it was just as I started to relax into my position on the bench that Coach hollered, "AJ, you're in!"

A full second ticked by as I sat there. And then another. And another. I sat wide-eyed and frozen until the tenth-grader next to me elbowed me hard in the ribs.

"You'd better go," she said.

I shot up and jogged stiffly out onto the court, and the whistle blew, signaling the game to resume. I played awkwardly and hesitantly. On defense, I guarded my opponent like my life depended on it. While on offense, I made sure to avoid the ball at all costs, not get in anyone's way. Yet despite these efforts, the ball was suddenly passed to me—and I caught it. I was immediately fouled. The ball was ripped out of my hands, and I was ushered over to the free-throw line. Players from both teams hurried to flank the sides of the key in front of me. It was all happening too fast. I had no time to process any of it as the referee tossed the ball back my way, and all the eyes in the entire gymnasium turned to me.

It was ghostly silent.

I rushed into it. Vibrating with nerves, I threw the ball up much too quickly, needing to get those eyes off of me. I missed the shot, wincing as the basketball clanged distastefully against the rim. The sound echoed embarrassingly in the following silence.

I breathed out a deep sigh, frustrated with myself. There wasn't any reason why I should have missed that shot, considering I'd won the citywide Knights of Columbus Free-Throw Championship every year. But the referee was already passing the ball to me for my second attempt; there was no time to dwell on any of that.

I received the bounce pass only a second later. Yet as my hands closed around the basketball this time, I felt something click. This was my moment. It wasn't the shy and uncertain Amelia standing there on the free-throw line with all those eyes trained on her. It was AJ. It even said so on the roster.

I took a deep breath, and I started my routine. The routine I'd rehearsed a thousand times.

I lined up my feet properly, taking the time to place my right foot slightly ahead of my left, the toe of my Nike only an inch behind the line. I bounced the ball once, instantly calming myself. Spun it only a single time in my hands, feeling the familiar pebbled leather whirl across my palms. I bounced it a second time. Bent my knees and took focus at the net. Tucking my right elbow and placing my hands in their practiced position along the seams, I exhaled and released.

The ball arched high, and everything was silent—all eyes watching, breaths held, players frozen. Time stood still. Then the ball swished perfectly through the exact center of the strings, making the most beautiful, flawless sound.

It was transformative—that single shot—the moment in which I became a real basketball player, scoring a point in a high school game when I was only eleven years old.

Dance would always have a small place in my heart, but it was clear it no longer suited me. Basketball had just solidified that. I would only go on to dance to complete my obligation for that year, as basketball became my passion. My addiction.

I was certain of where I belonged.

BEYOND

I am sitting naked, wrapped only in a towel, on the cold tile of the bathroom floor—still wet from my soak in the tub. I'm lightheaded, dizzy, and nauseated, and my heart is pounding out of control.

It's a terrible thing to be chronically cold yet intolerant to heat; a wicked cycle to go through all day. Freezing cold, warm bath, dizzy and nauseous. Freezing cold, warm bath, dizzy and nauseous. Over and over. But I have sixty-five symptoms now, so I don't have the energy to get too fussed about that.

For four hundred fifty-five days straight, I've had incapacitating chest pain that has prevented me from being able to sit, stand, or lie comfortably. For three hundred eighty-eight days now, I've not been able to speak more than the odd word, smile, or chew. I go to bed every single night with a migraine, toss and turn in the night with a migraine, and wake every morning with the exact same migraine. And I have to keep my phone on me at all times as a panic button in case I need to text for help, since I live each moment on edge, waiting for the electric pain attacks that drop me to the floor.

But I guess that's all old news.

Cognitively, my newest struggle is trying to count to five. I know logically the numbers that are supposed to come between one and five, yet for some reason, when I try to say them in order in my head, I get lost at three each time.

I've started hallucinating, too—so that's also new. It's never anything funny or entertaining, unfortunately, mostly just confusing and a bit alarming. Words rise up and dance on the page in front of me, and shapes and shadows appear out of nowhere. I find myself physically recoiling from them, swatting at the air, and throwing my arms up in front of me protectively. But the attack is always in my peripheral. When I turn my head to try to see it more clearly, it is there one second, and gone the next.

I've developed a tremor, an internal vibration deep inside my torso that, at times, occurs only on my left side. An external convulsion also starts in my right hand, and it slowly overtakes my entire body until even my teeth chatter along with it.

I have constant fasciculations, too, twitches like the small flutter of a butterfly trapped underneath my skin. They're incessant, going on for hours and days and weeks at a time, sometimes even months at a time. While that's undoubtedly unnerving, it is the violent muscle spasms that scare me the most. Like the one we think dislocated my jaw.

And I never even knew there could be so many different types of pain—a vast variety of sensations that all fall under that same generic umbrella term. Nor did I ever imagine that someone would have to endure all of those types of pain, all at the same time, every single day. But now I do.

I have arthritis all throughout my body; the worst of it in my knees, my hips, and my hands. The joints feel as if they are filled with concrete, heavy and stiff, and at times, they're locked, nearly immobile.

My heels, my fingertips, my left forearm, and my right thigh are constantly numb. I have three areas on my body that sting intensely and incessantly while surface-level sparklers dance randomly across my skin.

I often feel I have a severe sunburn, when I haven't been exposed to the sun in months. It seems I'm burning from the inside out, yet still, I'm hopelessly cold. And my entire body itches, at times, for days on end. I have to soak in a bathtub of baking soda even though I have no visible rash. The itching, too, seems to come from within.

There is a deep ache, especially in my tailbone and pelvis; my skeleton is simply too tender for furniture now. A boring neurogenic pain unrelentingly consumes my left thigh. A sharp, permanent stabbing lives in the muscle near my belly button (specifically at eleven o'clock). The area of pain is only the size of a dime, but is so sharp it takes my breath away. And a perfectly straight line of fire angles down from the right side of my ribcage to my pubic bone, which keeps me doubled over at all times.

An intense constricting pressure wraps around my lower ribs and upper abdomen as if I'm wearing a corset that is much, much too tight. I constantly adjust my posture in an attempt to escape it, and I struggle to breathe or eat.

My right calf pulses with a restrictive dysesthesia, like an invisible belt is tied too tightly around it, too. I worry my calf might burst from the pressure, and yet it simultaneously tingles. The sensations are confusing, achy, uncomfortable, and odd. I find myself neurotically researching compartment syndrome and checking it for signs of clots.

Sharp, lacerating, lancinating pains dominate the soles of my feet, and the bones all ache as though they have been broken. The touch of socks or bedsheets is intolerable, but anything is better than standing on the sharp shards of broken glass that have become my floor. I constantly look with a flashlight to see where my feet might be cut or where a tiny metal sliver could be embedded, yet I never find anything there.

My Achilles tendon feels torn. Whiplash prevents me from turning my head to either side. And sometimes, completely out of the blue, I get a stabbing pain far up inside of me. It is deep inside my vagina, up near my cervix; it can go on for ten minutes at a time as I twitch and writhe, whimper and contort. The pain penetrates me over and over again, like I'm being raped by a steak knife.

It seems there is no place in my body left untouched by this "Lyme."

And then there are the incidents, so many incidents, like what happened to me the other day. My husband had helped me out of bed and into the kitchen, and I was sitting at the island, a bowl of pureed soup he'd warmed in the microwave in front of me.

I was enjoying the change of scenery from being stuck in my bed, even if the sunlight was too bright coming through the windows. We sat there, slowly eating our lunch together in a serene, comfortable, and complete silence (we never have sounds in the house anymore; no TV, no music ever plays in the background). But just as I swallowed another spoonful of my soup, a gunshot rang out.

Instant pain shot through my ears, and my hands flew up instinctively to cover them. I burst into terrified tears. I trembled, holding my head between my hands as I started to rock back and forth. I tried to retreat into myself as terror raced through me; my heart rate and breathing were completely erratic. When finally the confusion caught up with me, I slowly opened a single eye to see what had happened.

And I saw it.

I had dropped my own spoon, and it had fallen with a clatter.

There was no gunshot. Yet there I was, acting like a veteran with post-traumatic stress disorder. My reaction was likely some result of being stuck in fight-or-flight mode, we later presumed, as for the last fifteen months, I've existed solely on a foundation of anxiety and panic. I've been consumed by this instinct, an innate knowledge that I'm not okay.

Probably because I'm not.

An invisible war rages inside of me. My bloodwork continues to worsen each month, as my organs aren't tolerating the treatment. My liver and kidneys ache deeply. I am ill with methemoglobinemia, a potentially fatal blood disorder that means my body is not getting enough oxygen. And my pure black stools are apparently a sign of an upper gastrointestinal bleed.

For the most part, I handle all of that. I handle sixty-five symptoms. The only thing that scares me, I mean, truly terrifies me, is still my very first symptom. It continues to attack in just two places—two completely different locations, yet somehow, I know they are the same.

The electrocutions in my face and in my heart.

I hadn't experienced such pain before, it is a severity I never even knew was possible. For over a year those electrocutions have been teaching me what *real* pain feels like—showing me the true extent of what pain can be—and I've become obsessed with needing an explanation.

I still struggle to believe that a hypothetical Lyme could be causing all of this. I worry the attacks in my face and in my chest are a sign of some internal failure, something that we shouldn't be trying to ignore or handle at home alone. I'm afraid that someday, one of these attacks will finally kill me because I was trained to suffer through—knowing that the hospitals were all unable and unwilling to help. But I don't get the impression the Lyme-guy wants to listen to my symptoms or theories anymore. Rather than give me any type of explanation for my pain, he continues to shrug and write it all off as "Lyme."

And I'm just not buying that.

"Where is this pain coming from?" my husband asked the Lyme-guy again this week at our December appointment.

"Tick-borne illness is known to cause pain," he replied in his usual flat monotone.

"Right, but how? Like, what's physically happening inside her body?" my husband kept trying. "Is something *else* wrong?"

"I assume she's had all the tests and scans your previous doctors could think of."

"Well, yeah…" my husband said, still talking for the both of us as I nodded along emphatically. "Maybe there are other tests, more tests that you know of."

This was met with silence. A shrug from the Lyme-guy, a slight purse of his lips.

"Could it be something other than Lyme?" my husband probed.

"Sure, in fact, it's probably *not* Lyme," the Lyme-guy replied with sudden enthusiasm, as if excited he had an answer for us.

My heart soared.

"It's probably *Babesia*."

My heart sank. I didn't get why this Lyme-guy always had to be such a purist. *Babesia, Bartonella, Borrelia,* it was all the same thing. Did he really not understand what we were asking?

"No, I mean another disease altogether," said my husband.

"Oh. Haven't you had testing for other diseases?" The Lyme-guy asked, now sounding both deflated and a bit confused.

"Well, yeah. Of course, she has."

"Okay."

"We're asking what's causing her pain?"

"Probably *Babesia.*"

"Right, but how?" my husband asked again, now going around in circles. "What's physically happening, structurally, or biologically inside her body to cause such pain?"

"Some of it could also be *Bartonella.*"

"Is it going to KILL me?" I blurted out through my broken jaw and mask, fed up with the nonsense.

Silence.

A few awkward seconds passed as we watched the Lyme-guy decipher those mumbled words and consider my question. He was never one to jump to conclusions or say anything too definitively, and I could see him processing outcomes in his mind, weighing all the options. He always chose his words carefully, as if he was trying to protect himself—from what, I never knew.

"Probably not?" The Lyme-guy eventually finished with a bit too much inflection in his voice for my liking. Then we all sat there in his office, the three of us considering that.

I wondered if the Lyme-guy maybe didn't get it; the story my husband had just told him was perhaps too unfathomable. But I feared that wasn't the case.

I was afraid he understood it all perfectly.

It came out of nowhere. We were sitting in our living room when I stopped breathing, lost all awareness, and cried out—first a high-pitched yelp and then a series of strangled moans gurgled out from deep inside me. My eyes rolled back into my head, and I could no longer see. My body fell onto our living room rug, grasping at my chest, writhing and contorting.

My back arched involuntarily as if electrified by the current, and I tried to twist away. I tried to escape it. Tears mixed with sweat, and my body spasmed as I was electrocuted over and over again. I whimpered in thirty-second intervals, the strangled mewing sounds coming out of me more like those of a dying animal than of anything human.

The pain may have started in my chest, but the live wire seemed to connect directly to my brain—somewhere behind my eyes. It had stunned me into nothingness. Erased any thoughts, sights, or sounds.

I should have been used to this type of pain, as it happened multiple times a day. Yet each time was so severe, so incapacitating, that there really was no *getting used to it*. All I'd been able to do this past year was settle into a rhythm with it, somehow learning for my own self-preservation when it was time to let go. I'd taught myself how to survive, how to find reprieve—how to black out.

So I stopped fighting it. I surrendered to the pain, and I let it take me.

I disappeared. Slipping away from my destructive physical body and into the inky darkness, my mind went blank, a bit like drifting off to sleep or fainting. Taken from a state of super-heightened awareness to a state of none, I went *beyond* the pain to a place where there was nothing at all.

It was neither warm nor cold, I looked around and found I was in darkness. There was only silence. There was nothing there. There was no pain, no fear; in this place, I simply existed.

I stayed there as if someone had hit pause on me. Time passed, but I was not aware of it. I was not aware of anything outside of *the beyond*. In here, everything for me was frozen.

In a way, it was beautiful—my reprieve—this place I'd created where I could go to survive. This place where fear and pain and even time did not exist.

At some point though, out of my own volition, I started to reenter my body. I was disappointed to find myself regaining consciousness again, wishing I could have stayed in *the beyond* for a little while longer.

I found myself exhausted and thoroughly drained, as it all rushed back at me. I was aware of everything again. The pain. The fear. My collapsed position on our walnut floor. The streams of tears that must have run down my face, leaving wet stains all over my clothing. And my husband crouched beside me, fear and concern etched over his beautiful face.

He handed me painkillers, and I swallowed them, with neither of us saying a word—we both knew the drugs wouldn't work, they never did. With my nod of permission, he reached for me and carried me to the bed.

He, too, would never be *used to this*, but we had our routine.

As he laid me on the bed to rest, however, the next shockwave instantly hit. I simultaneously prayed for healing or death, either one as long as the pain ended. But this time, it happened too quickly, and I couldn't escape into the darkness. I couldn't escape into my *beyond*.

This time, as my body lit up with the electricity, I saw the flash of light—the path and the intensity of the pain were so specific that my mind's eye actually saw it.

It was organically shaped, not dissimilar to a tree.

The ignition point started deep and red within my chest, a jolt of electric pain within the center of my heart. And immediately, it started to branch out three-dimensionally throughout my thoracic cavity.

Yellow flames began to course along the boughs, and I not only felt but *saw* each of those burning branches of pain. I weathered each dip and curve as the electric current flowed down the individual stems—the glowing yellow light following the offshoots as they forked off, subdividing into branchlets, and dividing again into twigs. It overtook my entire torso until the last of the little yellow flames reached the very tip of every single sprig, leaving the totality of my trunk on fire.

Then, a blinding flash of bright white.

BASKETBALL

THIRTEEN YEARS OLD

The summer before high school, I lived in my favorite orange and lime green tank top. My lanky arms were dark from the sun. My long blonde hair had been spritzed with lemon juice to make it a shade or two lighter. I'd sprouted up to five foot eight that year and had yet to reach a hundred pounds; I was thin, gangly, even. However, I found my athletic legs to be a bit disproportionate to the rest of my lithe body, and so I insisted on keeping them hidden. Much to my mother's disappointment, I completed my summer look by refusing to wear anything but my extra-wide-leg skater jeans—regardless of the outside temperature.

I thought the low-rise, oversized jeans and the tiny tank suited my daily skater girl look. I often wore backward hats and toques, even in the summer, to keep my hair out of my face. That suited the look, too. It was 1997, after all.

I'd finally found my confidence, popular with multiple groups of friends and a style of my own. I was a teenager with zero responsibilities, a mountain bike, and the freedom and independence to enjoy it all. I had the world by its tail (or at least the city of Moose Jaw), and I liked to spend every one of the long summer days riding around town with my friends.

We rode to different neighborhoods, visiting and collecting girls as we went. Our little bike gang grew in size at each subsequent stop. I liked swinging by Grandma Johnson's for a Pepsi and a slice of cold pizza and then to the corner store where we'd wander the aisles trying to decide between a Twix, Crunchie, or Mars. Though we usually settled on Slurpees and little plastic baggies filled with five-cent gummies—blue whales, frogs, fuzzy peaches, and Dino-Sours.

We'd borrow the extra waterski rope that hung in our garage and hook it up to the back of one of the bikes—one person pedaling as fast as she could as the rest of us took turns being pulled on our Rollerblades. We tried, completely unsuccessfully, to master jumps like we saw in the X Games, and messed around (again, mostly unsuccessfully) with Jade's brother's skateboard.

We often hung out at my house, as I had a private space in the basement that my dad had built just for me. It had a pool table and ping-pong, and even a swing hung from the ceiling joists. We loved NSYNC and the Backstreet Boys and spent hours singing off-key while we tried to perfect their dance moves. We were quickly becoming obsessed with all things romance: boys, rom-coms, and those '90s boy band ballads. I even had my very first kiss with the boy next door.

It was an awkward attempt between two kids, neither of whom was ready, on the sidewalk between our parents' houses late one summer night. It took us a long while of uncomfortable conversation standing there in the dark shadows, both of us trying to get up the nerve, when finally Danny just counted aloud for us to both lean in.

"One, two, three..."

I closed my eyes and pursed my lips, as I'd seen it done in all the movies—but he led with his mouth open and his tongue hanging out. And his tongue, slippery and wet, entered my mouth before our lips could even touch.

I immediately recoiled, horrified at the intrusion. Flooded with equal parts disgust and embarrassment that I'd maybe done it all wrong, I didn't admit to him that it had been my first time. Instead, I let him count us down again to try once more, yet the second our mouths met, it was exactly the same. I couldn't help but instantly pull away.

I tried to play it cool as I mumbled some fabricated excuse, claiming I needed to get back inside to where my friends were waiting for me. But the truth was, I couldn't wait to rinse my mouth out with Scope.

I'd only ever felt anxiety about two things in my life: as a young kid learning for the first time about the birds and the bees and anything medical. Both had seemed so incredibly gross. But that cringeworthy kiss triggered the return of those anxious feelings in me, and the memory of my humiliation stayed in the back of my mind, haunting me for the entire next year.

I avoided Danny. I tried to avoid boys altogether. Tried, of course, being the operative word—as no matter how hard I tried, by fifteen, I was no longer a stranger to receiving attention from boys.

I wished it could have been different. I wished *I* could have been different—like the girls I watched in all those rom-coms, who fell recklessly in love without a care in the world. Yet reality was turning out nothing like those movies.

I didn't feel any butterflies as boys asked me out, handing me one beautiful bundle of red roses after another on Valentine's. I felt nothing but awkwardness and uneasiness at the attention as I turned each of them down. Those bouquets, combined with the sweet roses my dad had delivered to the school for me each year, just meant I had a lot of flowers to try and hide in my locker. And that didn't go unnoticed.

My friends teased me mercilessly, sardonically referring to my group of male friends as the "AJ Fan Club." I found it embarrassing, not only for myself but also on behalf of the boys. Those guys were my friends, after all, and I didn't think it was fair that they should be mocked for their generosity and expression when it was obviously I who had the problem. I felt bad about it. The last thing I wanted was to hurt someone; I just knew I couldn't make myself feel something that I didn't. I still wasn't ready.

The most persistent of all the boys at the time was Cole. He was barely two inches taller than I, skinny yet athletically muscular in that way only young teenage boys could be. Though at best, he was only average-looking. I wasn't attracted to him.

He was always trying too hard—to look cool, dress the right way, act the right way. He even tried to listen to the right music in the right way—driving too fast around town in his black convertible, blasting Eminem with the bass turned up. He needed to be popular. Needed to be a part of the *in* group. But sadly, he was always precariously right on the fringe (almost in, yet at any moment, he could be out), and that threat only seemed to reinforce his need to keep trying so hard.

I didn't find his desperation attractive.

He was even always trying too hard to get *me* to like him. He'd had a crush on me for over a year and had been unabashedly persistent despite my unreciprocated interest. He'd called incessantly, loitered in the gym to offer me a ride home after practice, and for two years in a row, he'd been one of those boys who gave me flowers on Valentine's.

Everywhere I turned, Cole was there waiting for me.

I found it annoying.

However as the months passed, despite the jock bravado he'd always insisted on having in front of everyone else, he started to let me see the real him. And I discovered, underneath his tough facade, that he was actually a good guy. He was kind and sweet, and slowly, he worked his way into my life, becoming my friend.

Cole wasn't satisfied with being my friend. His chase remained intense—continually, exasperatingly, relentless. Embarrassing even. Though maybe the odd time, I did find it flattering, even if I wasn't interested in him romantically at all.

I had a crush on his friend Tyler, but I'd been too shy on our one and only attempt at a date. I hadn't been comfortable. Just as I'd been too timid with other boys I'd previously had crushes on, I was too afraid to put myself out there with Tyler, too afraid to go after a guy I actually liked. I was new to dating, and I needed assurance.

Cole gave that to me. As time passed and I grew up and matured, I found Cole was still there, still waiting for me, and I could no longer remember the reasons for my earlier trepidations. He'd been good to me all that time, kind and respectful, and I was comfortable with him—

knowing that he was just as insecure and inexperienced as I was. I'd even come to like having him around; his presence helped quell some of the unwanted attention from other boys, giving my anxiety a chance to fade away. And agreeing to date Cole suddenly seemed easier than continuing to turn him down. I didn't want to hurt his feelings any longer.

Besides, we had sports in common. It was about as simple as that.

I even grew to love Cole, just as I loved each of my friends. I loved every aspect of being in high school—the way my world was expanding, the gained friendships, the extracurriculars, the more complex classes. But above all, my true love was always basketball. I lived in the Vanier Collegiate gym.

I practiced with three different teams that year: the VCI junior team, the senior team, and even the boys team let me practice with them daily. I started most of my days around six a.m., with a practice before classes even began. During the lunch break, I shot hoops and studied plays—excited to join two more teams after school for two full-on back-to-back practices.

I was a gym rat, and I absolutely loved it.

It was my dream to play in the WNBA; the league was new, and it was all I could think about. I started working extra hard, practicing my vertical, perfecting my ball-handling skills, and sitting on the kitchen counter talking strategy late into the evenings with my dad. And with my sole focus on basketball, I avoided anything that would risk my chance of succeeding.

I didn't skip school, and I made sure to get straight A's. I didn't smoke, drink, or do drugs at parties, and I never missed my curfew. Instead, I read all of the basketball magazines I could get my hands on, had NBA posters pinned up all over my room, and I played every season in the latest Air Jordans. Even my first jobs were all basketball-related.

I worked part-time at Foot Locker in the mall, unintentionally earning the job one day when the general manager overheard me talking enthusiastically about sneakers. He'd walked right up to me and offered me a job on the spot. And Coach A hired me as the manager of the

Vanier scorekeepers, in addition to training me as a referee. He even set up a camp for elementary school kids, which we coached together on the weekends.

Gone was the eleven-year-old kid who avoided the ball like her life depended on it. I wanted the ball, had a hunger for the ball, and an insatiable hunger for the sport. And maybe for the first time ever, with JJ off at university, I felt like I was living my own life—no longer a follower, but maybe a bit like a rock star myself. Especially during games like the one we played against Riverview.

The energy was high, the gym lights bright, and the boisterous sounds of the crowd, the coaches' calls, and squeaking sneakers reverberated around the gym. We were winning in those first few minutes of the second half, but not by a lot.

We were on defense, and I was loosely guarding my opponent just outside the three-point line, hanging back to see as much as I could with my peripheral. Caitlyn, Melanie, and the posts were down in the key, and Sarah and Leah and their girls were out in the wings with the ball.

Just as Riverview passed up top, I saw my opportunity.

I lunged forward, my fingertips barely grazing the ball, knocking it ahead of me as I rushed after it. Claiming it, regaining control. My long legs burst down the court as I left everyone else behind and successfully made an easy layup.

Cole, my parents, and the crowd cheered, and there were high fives all around as I jogged back to take my place on defense again. But I wasn't celebrating. I was focused. My opponent, Riverview's point guard, was bringing the ball down the court once more.

She approached me, ball-handling with her left this time, and as I put a little pressure on her, she crossed to her right, pointing and calling out plays to her teammates behind me as she went. "Number three, number three, down low."

She was distracted. I reached in and cleanly stole the ball from her—her dribbling becoming mine—the rhythm hardly broken in the exchange. And as I sprinted down the court toward my own basket, I saw that only the power forward from Riverview had kept pace with me. I approached the top of the key, faked like I was going to continue right, and then made a quick behind-my-back to my left to lose her. I dribbled once, stopped short, went up, and sank a little jump shot with my left hand.

My face was red with excitement and exertion as I jogged back to take my place on defense, with whoops from my team and the crowd all around. Riverview was rattled, and it was starting to show, but I knew *I* was just getting started.

Within seconds, my opponent was bringing the ball up the court, and I hung back loosely yet again. Though the second she went to bounce pass it to her forward, I lunged in and stole it—the third time in only three possessions.

My team followed me down the court toward our net, and seeing this, rather than score myself, I paused and passed the ball to Sarah. She was a sweet girl who only ever played in the shadows. I'd watched her work hard in practice, but knew she never saw much action during the games.

Sarah froze, clearly unsure what to do at having received the ball. She just stared at me, wide-eyed and stunned until I ran over and set a quick screen for her.

"Go!" I directed. And as I rolled, turning out of the pick, I watched as she dribbled once, took the choreographed steps she had practiced so many times before, and made the layup. Immediately turning back to me, I saw her face was bursting with excitement.

"Yes!" she cried as the team rushed in to give her high fives. And the game went on like that.

I stole the ball about a dozen times during that final half, not only making several more shots myself but sharing the action with all of my team's underdogs. I left the gym with a sense of satisfaction that day—though not because we had won, and not because I had led the team in points, steals, and assists, which I often did. But more importantly, it had been fun to see Sarah's look of surprise at having received the ball, and it had melted my heart to see her joy at scoring.

That game had been a success for all of us, and in that, I'd felt the true significance of what it meant to be a part of a team. Basketball had transformed me, from a shy and uncertain girl so quiet her teachers could barely hear her, into a powerful and confident athlete. A team captain and a leader.

I truly had it all.

KRISTIN

SEVENTEEN YEARS OLD

I was sitting in the passenger seat of Coach's sedan as he drove me home after our tournament, proudly wearing my medal and chatting enthusiastically nonstop. When just as he turned the final corner onto my street, I stopped speaking mid-sentence.

JJ's car was in our driveway.

I hadn't expected her home from university that weekend, and a flush of excitement washed over me upon seeing that little red Celica in its usual spot. I jumped out of Coach's car with a quick "thanks," slammed the door, and jogged up the sidewalk to our house.

I came to an immediate halt when I saw JJ standing there, waiting for me in the foyer. Her expression was somber, and we didn't really *do* somber.

Before I could ask, JJ stepped toward me without saying a word. She simply wrapped me in her arms—holding me while I stood awkwardly confused.

There was a brief pause.

"Kristin died today."

All the air left my body as I collapsed into her.

There was an even longer pause.

"I won my tournament," I finally managed to whisper back.

I hadn't seen it coming.

Of course, I'd known that Kristin was sick, but I never could understand it.

My life had been fairly simple. I'd continued to excel both in school and at sports, despite sustaining a tear in my knee playing fastball and a minor corrective surgery. I had several best friends, my boyfriend Cole, and no desire to be any more popular than that. Getting along with most everyone at school—the athletes, the nerds, and the cool kids alike—I was comfortable in all areas of my life.

At times, I felt guilty about that.

I sometimes wondered if I'd become a self-absorbed teenager, wrapped up in the all-consuming world that was high school. But maybe I simply couldn't compute the injustice of it all, that my baby cousin had been forced to endure something so awful. Either way, it was a testament to my parents for sure, that despite the fear rippling through our family at that time, they'd managed to ensure my final semesters could still be so great.

I'd been told that Kristin had some type of virus attack her lymph nodes, but she'd gotten better within the month. Taking swimming lessons in the winter, soccer in the summer, and always talking a mile a minute, I could see that nothing was going to hold that girl back. She was exuberant. And super smart, too—she was enrolled in the advanced enrichment program at École St. Margaret. She loved school, loved her friends and family. She loved everything.

Then she got sick again, rushed into the ICU in Regina one day when her kidneys failed. I'd watched Kristin's blonde hair fall out after that. The transition from long to short to a perfectly smooth and shiny scalp, and I'd gone immediately to the mall with my mom to buy her some hats. But she reached what they called remission fairly quickly, so it had truly never crossed my adolescent mind that she wouldn't be okay.

She was sick again by that December, and while I welcomed in the new year with Cole, surrounded by all of our friends, Kristin welcomed it in from a bed in the ICU. Yet, I still didn't see it coming.

Especially not on the day Mom and I drove Kristin and Auntie Mary home from the hospital. I was at the wheel with Kristin beside me, and our moms were in the back. And just as my mom had always done with me, I cranked the music up a bit too loud.

The sun was shining, and I felt a sense of freedom cruising down the open prairie highway, singing away with Kristin to my newest CD of '90s pop tunes. Everything was going to be okay now; we were driving away from the hospital, away from the darkness and into the light. We were leaving her illness and all of our troubles behind. And even though we didn't talk about it, I sensed Kristin was feeling that exact same way.

She looked at me and smiled, probably not dissimilar to how I'd always looked at JJ, and I felt a complete sense of warmth and contentedness in that moment. In our shared look. My heart was brimming with love as I smiled back at her—both of us dancing in our seats to the music, the sun sparkling all around.

That moment, that look, both perfect—frozen forever in my mind. I just knew everything was going to be okay.

She had a bone marrow transplant that summer, and Mom, Auntie Janet, and I drove into Winnipeg to see her. And yet again, Kristin was doing really well. She was less active—with chess, board games, and arts and crafts, her new pastimes—but her joy and her light had never dimmed. She was, as always, the brightest light in our family.

Even when her Make-A-Wish was granted that fall, I still wasn't sure I understood its implications. Although I definitely should have clued in when we celebrated her twelfth birthday, nearly six months before her actual birthday.

My mom sat me down in advance of that party and explained that it was unlikely Kristin would make it to August. Kristin had even had a dream about it—a premonition regarding her passing in which she wore a crown. I was to be prepared that she would be wearing a crown at her party, too. But even as my mom told me all of that, it didn't feel real.

I attended the party at her house that weekend with a fake smile plastered on my face. For once, I was completely uncomfortable in the familiar living room—unsure what to say or what to believe about Kristin's timeline, when everything about the gathering appeared otherwise so normal. Our family all together as we usually were. The immense amount of food spread out on the dining room table: Grandma's homemade buns, a charcuterie board and vegetable tray, chips, multiple dips, and spreads. All of our favorites. There was even birthday cake, balloons, and laughter all around me. Yet, I felt so out of place.

I stuffed these emotions down, refusing to cry in front of Kristin while she managed to sit there so calmly, seemingly unfazed by her own mortality at only eleven years old. I tried to follow the lead of my other family members, even if it didn't feel right to do so six months too early.

"Happy Birthday," I told her cautiously as I approached.

She smiled, looking up at me from her special chair and with a crown on her head. "It's a little early, but I won't be here in August."

My breath caught—she'd said it so easily, as if she was simply planning on being away on vacation or something. Though I knew that's not at all what she'd meant.

She'd even managed to look happy in that moment, surrounded by all of our family. But I recognized that she wore that smile in part to comfort us, and it was that realization, above everything else, that was breaking my heart the most.

I couldn't get out of there soon enough.

I was working Hoopla that weekend (the provincial championship tournament for high school basketball), and I'd only been given a two-hour break to attend the party. I hated feeling rushed, but a part of me *was* grateful for the excuse to leave. Grateful to escape back to the normality of work. My sanctuary of the gym. The basketball court. Yet, relieved as I was to hurry back to the comfort of the gym, I had a niggling sense that I hadn't done enough for Kristin that day. I hadn't done enough for her during the years she'd been sick.

We'd spent our entire childhood growing up together, and I had always loved her like a little sister, truly never fathoming that our time could be limited. But now, for the first time ever, I wondered if maybe it would.

If that was the case, I hadn't done enough for her—period.

I just hadn't seen it coming. Even as she'd been fighting for her life, I'd only ever seen her youthful joy and the light in her eyes. I'd wholeheartedly believed she would be okay.

She was only eleven years old.

And eleven-year-old children are supposed to be okay.

I felt sick—still standing there in the foyer, with JJ wrapped around me. My team had been winning our tournament during the exact moment Kristin had died; and the dichotomy of those simultaneous events was too much for me to bear.

My body revolted.

More than sad, I was distraught. Destroyed. I threw up all week, couldn't bring myself to eat or sleep, and became a walking zombie. I was so physically ill that I couldn't even attend the family prayers at the church on Friday night.

Her death had rocked my idyllic little world.

Come Saturday morning, still throwing up, I had to force myself to attend the funeral. The first thing I noticed as I entered St. Joseph's church was that Kristin's casket was beautiful. A pure, glossy white.

Upon a closer look, however, I realized it was unnervingly small. Too small. It was, of course, a child's casket. And in the last remaining moments before the funeral was to start, in the grand foyer of the big, traditional Catholic church, our family gathered around it. Soft, natural sunlight streamed in through stained-glass windows, while that pristinely white, too-small casket glowed ethereally in the center of us all.

Each family member took a turn writing on the casket, messages of love and messages of goodbye. Though I'd been told in advance that this was what we would be doing, each writing our final words to her, I didn't feel prepared. My heart ached. I stood there at a loss as to what I could possibly write to summarize my love, my pride in her bravery, or my grief at her sudden disappearance. The emptiness that I now felt.

I took the marker solemnly as it was passed to me, and I looked down at the love-filled messages from each of my grief-stricken family members that already decorated the lid. They were all so beautiful—handwritten personal messages of love in black marker scripted across the glossy white. And my words, the only words I could think of, did not feel like enough.

You did good, Buddy.
I love you.

I didn't feel any better after having written those words. And as I numbly handed the marker off to JJ beside me, a wave of panic washed over me—I should have copied what my uncle had written. But I couldn't make sense of anything that was happening; time was moving too fast for me to keep up.

If those had been my final words to her, they hadn't been enough. Words were just words, after all, and even though I'd meant them with my entire heart, they would never be enough.

It was surreal that I wouldn't be seeing her again, and my grief was overwhelming me. It was gathered in the corners of my eyes and lodged like a lump in the back of my throat. My thoughts and emotions were stuck and unmoving, filling the hollow parts of my chest so completely that I felt sharp, physical pain as a result. I knew the pressure of all that building grief was causing my heart to crack the slightest bit. I could feel it erupting into tiny fissures, my emotions and lost words aching inside of me.

For self-preservation, I had to tune out the service. Nauseous as I was, I hung my head down the entire time. I stared unfocused at my stupid black tights instead, blocking out words and prayers and all other attendees around me, until eventually, the service was over, and I blindly followed JJ and Kyle to exit our pew.

I only looked up when I realized that it was Kristin's young classmates who were leading the way. I hadn't expected that. I hadn't noticed at all who'd been in attendance; I'd been merely surviving, one emotional blow after the next. And as I looked at them, taking in their presence for the very first time, I felt my heart break a little bit more upon seeing the young, grieving children.

I watched them as they led my family down the rich burgundy carpeted aisle past the darkly stained wooden pews. The grand arch of the domed ceiling towered above us while beams of sunlight still streamed in through the stained glass windows, softly lighting our way. But I never took my eyes off the children as they exited through the grand foyer and through the double wooden doors leading outside. They broke into two separate groups and formed two separate lines, as if in some sort of planned choreography. They only came to a stop once they were all standing formally, facing inwards, lining each side of the exit out of St. Joseph's church and down the grand exterior staircase.

Confusion, then realization, then horror dawned on me that *this* was a part of the procession. And that *we*, the family, were now expected to accompany the casket and walk between those two rows of sobbing children.

I wasn't sure if I could do it—but there was no other choice as my family continued on.

My dad and uncles led the way as pallbearers, carrying the white, too-small casket decorated with all of our handwritten goodbyes. The procession was both beautiful and heart-wrenching as my entire family followed behind—the children's sobs echoing ahead of us in the distance. Their grief seemed to come to a crescendo as we walked between the two rows, down the grand staircase and pathway, and toward the waiting limousines. And it was then, with the sounds of the crying children reverberating all around me, that my fractured heart broke all the way open.

My sobs joined in their symphony.

MISUNDERSTOOD

Sometimes I find myself hoping that I have a different disease. Like, if I have to be this sick, why can't I at least have something less controversial? Something believable. Recognizable, with medical support. Something that would speak for me so that I won't always have to.

Lyme disease has been called "the infectious disease equivalent of cancer," yet few people seem to know that. Few people know much about Lyme disease at all, in fact, but everyone knows what cancer is. You don't have to waste what little strength you have explaining, justifying, and defending when you have cancer. Trying to convince those around you—friends, family, and trained medical professionals alike—that cancer is real.

Simply trying to convince yourself that cancer is real.

We might be surrounded by large, beautiful hospitals all throughout our city, yet when they think you have Lyme disease, you know those hospitals aren't meant for you. I've been there. They don't believe, recognize, or treat that illness, and they certainly don't know how to help a Herxing patient (not that your insurance would cover your time there anyway). Those of us suspected to have Lyme have already learned there is no comparative level of care.

The two diseases may be scientifically similar in many ways, but not in how our society reacts to them. There is a reverence for cancer, an understanding in society, whereas for Lyme, there is none.

When someone gets cancer, prayers and meals are offered—not unsolicited medical advice and opinions. No one blames the cancer on anxiety. No one accuses the patient of exaggerating or of having a poor attitude. And no one suggests the person with cancer isn't trying hard enough to get better, or suggests they should forgo treatment altogether—instead, simply believing their way into remission.

Rather, through chemo, their bald head becomes a neon-flashing sign announcing their illness, and their strength is applauded. But with Lyme treatment, there is no neon sign. Your strength, your struggle, is not recognized. The severity of your illness even gets dismissed as you are repeatedly told, "You look fine," "You don't look sick," "You look good, though." When people should know that illness is rarely something that the outside person can see.

I might look "fine"—but I am not.

I've kept most of my hair, but I've lost nearly everything else. Lost my independence and my ability to walk. Lost my smile. Lost my ability to communicate, both with my words and facial expressions. I've lost my ability to connect. My humanness. My personality. My sense of self. Yet I am continually told, "At least it's not cancer."

Now, obviously, I don't *want* to have cancer—I don't want to have any horrific disease at all. My point is that just because cancer is the big one we hear about the most in the media, it doesn't mean that all other diseases are less valid. Or less severe. With those types of comments, people are missing the fact that I'm already that sick. I *am* cancer-level sick. I fight every single day to survive, yet because our only "good" theory at this point is Lyme disease, I've received hardly any support—medical or otherwise. Doctors, friends, and extended family alike still don't seem to understand the brutality of what I am facing.

I don't want a neon sign.

But I would like to feel seen.

While I initially felt obligated to tell my friends and family I was ill, many of those earlier conversations didn't go well for me, and I regretted sharing about it at all. Their responses were indifferent, detached. Some replies were overall unconcerned, and a few were even flippant. More than one person surmised that they, too, "could have Lyme," despite not having any symptoms themselves. Others expressed disbelief, invalidating the seriousness of my illness and dismissing my fears. They questioned that my jaw had actually been dislocated and that it still was months later. They questioned that I was in pain every single day. They questioned that I was in pain during the very conversation we were having.

I received a lot of toxic positivity in lieu of actual support, platitudes like, "It could be worse," "Just think positively," and even, "You'll get over it." They sent me inspirational quotes with phrases like, "Life is short" and "Carpe diem" which only highlighted the fact that they didn't understand at all what I was going through, as it's awfully hard to "seize the day" when you keep blacking out from pain.

Even old people didn't seem to get it. As random strangers in waiting rooms went out of their way to tell me, "Just wait until you get older," they completely missed the irony that they were walking better than I was, forty years their junior. And at the rate I'm going, I might not ever get the chance.

When I texted a few close friends to admit that I felt disconnected, I was told, "Everyone feels that way because of the pandemic." Now I'm not going to claim to understand how everyone has felt during COVID, but it would be my guess that not everyone out there is completely bedridden, unable to work or drive themselves anywhere, and on top of it all, is unable to speak due to a dislocated jaw. It would be my guess that I'm a bit more disconnected than most.

Yet through all of this, a few of my neighbors, who had had a front-row seat to my decline, still continued to text me for favors like babysitting, feeding their dog, or watering their plants. "Seeing as you're home anyway," they texted, "maybe you could pop over?"

And it's not that I'm looking for sympathy here.

But I would like to feel heard.

I've had to decline a number of design jobs, writing back to explain that I'm not currently working due to illness. I even went so far as to clarify that I'm not capable of leaving the house, and that I'm unable to walk or even think clearly at the moment. Still, some people suggested they would "send pictures regardless. Unless you want to come take a look?" As if their projects were more important than my health.

While at my most recent MRI, upon hearing that I might have Lyme disease, the technician genuinely asked me if it was the "real" kind—as if there were some other. And in another attempt to find someone to reset my dislocated jaw (that *still* won't open), the brilliant advice I received from the esteemed doctor was to "not use straws or engage in oral sex."

What is wrong with people?

And how is it that they still don't understand?

I'm blown away by the amount of unwarranted medical advice random people have offered me, like suggestions that my pain is indigestion, and I should "try Rolaids." Or that I need to do more visualizations, more meditations, more yoga. More doctors. Different doctors. More medications. Less medications. Their words insinuate that I'm not better yet because I'm doing it wrong—or maybe I'm not trying hard enough. It depends on whom you ask; they all seem to have an opinion.

In response to my individual symptoms, I continually hear things like, "Oh yeah, I've had that." And in response to the possibility of Lyme, they say things like, "I think my mom had that," as if Lyme disease is something easy to overcome and just as easy to forget.

People love likening my situation to theirs, especially when they're down for a few days with a cold or a flu—as if our maladies are somehow the same. I've even been told that they understand what it's like not to be able to walk because they once "stubbed their toe quite severely."

It seems that everyone around me "understands" my situation. And though I try to tell myself that these comments are well intentioned, that people are trying to relate to me by attempting to normalize my illness, I don't need anyone to try and normalize seventy symptoms. There isn't anything normal about that.

I'm shutting down. I don't even want to disclose that I might have Lyme disease to the rest of my friends and family, and for those who already do know, I've learned to stop sharing the details. I've learned to avoid those who will just cause me additional anxiety, repeatedly questioning what it is that I'm doing. "Is it supposed to make you this sick?" "Why aren't you better yet?" "How come other people can heal their Lyme disease and you can't?" These questions trigger a fear that constantly haunts me.

I'm missing something.

This possible diagnosis—my treatment—still isn't correct.

I mean, being mysteriously ill is difficult enough, but having to deal with everyone's reactions to it absolutely drains me.

I try to be patient with their lack of understanding; it wasn't that long ago that I, too, didn't know this level of sick existed. In my limited past experience, sick people either got better, or they died. It hadn't occurred to me that there could be a third option. That someone could languish in the in-between—chronically—for years, even. Not living, but not dying either. Yet, even though I recognize that most people have little experience with chronic illness, it's hard not to be hurt when so many have stopped checking in. Even the few who'd initially handled my illness quite well have faded away, clearly not understanding the gravity of my "at least it's not cancer" situation.

Perhaps these people thought I got better, or maybe they forgot altogether that I was even sick, but I fear they simply gave up on me. As friends and family continue to dwindle away, stop checking in, and move on with their lives without me in them, I feel very forgotten. My entire world has shrunk, taking place in only two rooms of this house with only four people (my husband here, and JJ and my parents on the phone up in Canada). We have no visitors. The doorbell never rings, and neither does my cell. Even text messages are rare, and email is obsolete. I've been forced to acknowledge that many of my past relationships were pretty one-sided. Friends never hesitated to take from me when there was something that they needed, but now, in my time of need, I find myself very much alone.

I'm experiencing a level of sick that few will ever have to endure in their lives—an isolation and loneliness, a severity of pain that is worse than what most can even imagine. And I guess all I wanted was a text from them. A note to say, "I'm sorry" or "I'm thinking of you." A gesture to let me know that someone out there remembered me and cared. A few moments of their time, and perhaps someone to understand why I needed it so much.[2]

Instead, I've been trapped in this house, trapped in this bed, having to watch an entire lifetime of relationships disappear. Now too much time has passed. Too much has happened to me in their absence, so that if someone finally did reach out, I wouldn't even know how to respond.

Like: "How are you?"

I've been struggling to answer that for months.

I want to be honest, but the issue is that I've never been comfortable with negativity. I've never been sick before—I don't really know *how* to be a sick person—and I feel a pressure that I'm somehow doing it wrong. As if I'm supposed to be open and vulnerable while always remaining optimistic. Inspiring even. When that's not at all how I feel.

I'm not inspirational; I'm hopeless.

But I can't tell people that.

So I don't say much. I'm vague and evasive as I keep my walls up, hiding the extent of how I feel. Even though I ache inside for understanding, I know all those previous attempts only left me feeling even more disconnected. Now it feels too vulnerable, too exposed to open up about any of those things anymore. Even if this only compounds the problem, further exacerbating the misperception of how ill I truly am, I simply can't keep myself open to that type of heartache any longer.

Now, no interaction is normal for me anymore. Each one feels disingenuous, fake, and forced as I try to hide my anguish. I have feelings of guilt on top of it all that I had to push some people away—but I get the sense it would be inappropriate to tell my friends I think I'm dying, and worse yet, to tell them that I might like to. And I don't have a response for *how* I am right now because I'm not even sure *who* I am anymore.

I'm afraid that I may have permanently lost myself. That I will never again be who I once was. So when they ask an innocuous, "How are you?" I try not to let my eyes well up with tears, and I lie.

A deep loneliness cultivates there, in the seeds that are those lies. I might be trapped in this house and communicating via words on a screen, yet I know that loneliness doesn't stem from too much time spent alone but rather from being so profoundly misunderstood. I'm existing in a state that few can relate to—alive but not actually living. And with the silence from my friends and family so deafening, I think it is that loneliness of disconnection, not the disease itself, that's going to eventually destroy me.

"In suffering, I am unique and alone in the universe."[3] I know I can't change any of that. Only I can feel this pain. It is my lungs that struggle to breathe, my heart that struggles to beat, and my jaw that is too broken to speak—I will always be alone in all of that. But I can be prepared for the next time I am texted the very simple, yet very loaded, question, "How are you?" I won't be caught off guard again.

I've decided to tell them, "I'm working on healing." It's a simple line that I think should work; a response that aligns with my residual self-image, pleasant and polite, honest and optimistic. I think it should suffice.

Though it is underneath that scripted line that I will hide the full extent of my pain. Only I will know the truth. And I won't tell them, because they wouldn't understand it anyway, that another day has gone by that we didn't open the blinds. Another day I didn't get washed or dressed. And another day I spent crying in agony.

I'm starting to wonder if it was just another day lost to Lyme disease.

CHANGE

SEVENTEEN YEARS OLD

Two months after Kristin's passing, in June of 2001, I graduated high school at the top of my class, winning a handful of university scholarships. I didn't feel any nostalgia for leaving the familiar halls of Vanier behind; in fact, I couldn't wait to start the next chapter of my life. I was ready to move away. Ready to move on.

At JJ's suggestion for a summer job (she guessed I would enjoy working outdoors and with animals), I interviewed to be an interpreter at the Saskatchewan Burrowing Owl Interpretive Centre. Even though I had no idea what that job would entail.

The interview was held at the Moose Jaw Exhibition office, and after a successful forty-minute chat with Heath, the Centre's director, he pointed across the grounds to where I would spend my summer working. I nodded my head enthusiastically for his benefit—I was already vaguely familiar with the Moose Jaw Ex, having attended both the Hometown Fair and a few weddings in the Convention Centre there before. I'd just never noticed the few small buildings that stood in the distance, bordering the prairie pasture. But I smiled in understanding anyway, again for his benefit, as it all looked like it would suit just fine.

On my first day of work, I followed Heath's directions and parked my forest green Sunfire randomly on the gravel out front of one of those small buildings. It was no more than a tin shack, really, with a crooked and rusted sign on the door that read: *Office*.

I got out of my car and walked slowly toward it, suddenly trepidatious about the strange, caged area that encompassed the door. A screened-in porch would have been too polite of a description. The entire thing was rickety, built of raw lumber and wire mesh, like a bad do-it-yourself project.

A horse wandered over through the pasture to inspect what I was doing, and I cast a sideways glance in its direction. I raised a single eyebrow and shrugged a shoulder. Then I knocked on the outside door gently, hoping the entire thing wouldn't fall over. And I waited.

When no answer came, I glanced at the horse a final time and cautiously opened that first door to step inside the small, caged entrance—startling as the raw wood door slammed shut behind me. I took a deep breath and composed myself, strode forward two paces before I could think too much about it, and knocked on the second door.

"It's open," a voice called from inside.

I swallowed the lump in my throat, turned the handle, and stepped into the tiny space.

The first thing I noticed was that it was dark inside. The space was illuminated by only a single, bare bulb hanging overhead and a small window on the far left wall. I squinted in the dimness, my eyes not yet adjusted from the sunlight outside. I could just barely make out that the walls inside were tin—same as the exterior. However, as my eyes became accustomed, more came into focus. I absorbed the mess of random office furniture, filing cabinets, and stacks upon stacks of papers littering every surface. I tried not to react, tried not to look fazed by it all. Instead, I forced myself to make eye contact through the semidarkness with the few people sitting inside. Feigning confidence despite the disarray, and intent on looking competent for the start of my new job, I introduced myself. "Hey, I'm Amelia."

That's when the smell hit me.

It was musty, reminiscent of a dirty hamster cage, combined with the slight waft of damp hay and horse manure coming in through the small window. But the worst of it was the undeniable stench that something had indeed died, and its flesh was rotting somewhere over in the far corner. The lack of air conditioning wasn't helping the situation either. I'd never been in an "office" like that before.

Determined to remain poised and professional and trying not to trip on any of the boxes at my feet, I moved to shake the hand of the woman sitting closest to me.

Out of nowhere, a small bird flew at my head. I yelped and ducked out of the way as it narrowly missed me. The staff suppressed giggles at my reaction (or over-reaction), and I flushed red as a result. The reason for the caged entrance had made sense in my mind much too late.

Straightening to my full height and readjusting my shirt and ponytail, I worried I wasn't making the best first impression—not that this place was making the greatest impression on me either. With three long summer months looming in front of me, I worried I'd made a big mistake.

I wasn't sure what I'd gotten myself into.

Not long after that, I learned the Owl Centre was a new non-profit organization working on getting established (which explained why they had been using the old farm buildings already on the land and the overall shambles I'd found it all in).

I quickly came to adore the little owls, who stood barely taller than a pop can. I was saddened to hear that not only was there something called an endangered species list, but our precious burrowing owls were on it. This was the reason we were all there: the conservation of both the owls and their prairie habitat through education, stewardship, and ecotourism as our mission.

We would raise awareness about endangered species by giving tours and presentations, as well as help with research, bird-banding, and releasing owlets into the wild. While on-site, we would be responsible for caring for over a dozen rescued owls.

The little owls all looked more or less identical to each other, so I was taught to identify them by their nearly imperceptible differences, traits, and preferred perches. Spike was the darkest one in the enclosure, with the least amount of spots. Scamper was thinner; his mottled white feathers always laid a bit smoother than any of the others. And the one who'd nearly hit me in the head that first day was Luna, a domesticated/imprinted burrowing owl—the one I ended up getting to know the best.

We had a similar job description, she and I—working together to help educate the public, as she sat on my hand during each of those presentations I gave to tourists and school groups alike. It was out of my comfort zone (public speaking, that is), but having Luna on my hand alleviated some of the pressure. The schoolchildren didn't care much at all about what I was saying or if my voice faltered—like during the more difficult talks that I had to give in French. Everyone's eyes were always glued to that owl. And without fail, Luna pooped on my hand at some point during every one of those presentations, making the kids howl with laughter.

It was more than I could have ever hoped for my first full-time summer job. Even with the poop on the hand.

The staff was young, enthusiastic, and likable, and as the weeks and months passed, we worked alongside each other, bonding in our attempt to make something of the place. It was my first foray into construction, and I found I liked the challenge of a fixer-upper.

We remodeled a Quonset to house the displays, spraying down the moldy walls with bleach and then repainting. We redid the grounds, tediously planting native prairie plants across several acres. We even built a gazebo with a viewing platform and a thousand-foot-long barn-red fence encircling it all. We spent hours every day together, covered in dust and sweat. I loved it—loved being out in the sunshine, working with the birds, and bringing carrots to the horses in the neighboring pasture. I wasn't even grossed out that we had to feed the owls dead mice or that we were constantly covered in mysterious bug bites. The work felt valuable.

The work *was* valuable.

I happily spent my evenings and weekends hanging out with my high school friends and a new group from Peacock Collegiate. Ignoring

Cole's poor attitude and selfish desire to have me all to himself, I immersed myself in the joy of attending parties and late-night bonfires and making as many new friends as possible. I even took a few of my closest friends, Jade and Tara, on a girls' trip up to my beloved Waskesiu.

It felt like a summer of growth, and the months were flying by.

I couldn't believe it was already September, as I found myself in the family van with my mom and JJ, pulling onto the university campus. I tried to play it cool as my mom parked in the lot outside the dorms at the Language Institute and we all got out. I looked around at what would be my new home.

Wascana Park ran along the north side of the campus, where big oak trees stood tall above a walking path along the river. Native grasses blew in the wind along its banks. A single dragon boat glided across the waters. And a flock of Canada geese flew overhead in a perfect V-formation.

To the south stood the stone and brick academic buildings, which created a semi-circle around a giant green lawn. The historical buildings were certainly impressive in their grandeur, though I imagined the walls were also steeped with unknown wisdoms. I found the campus vibe overall intimidating; as students lounged and played frisbee, they somehow exuded both equal parts swag and cerebral.

It's not that I hadn't been there many times before, in the three years while JJ was a student, but the campus now looked different to me. I picked up my suitcase with nervous excitement, turning back to my mom when the significance of the moment finally hit.

"Be safe, okay?" she said. "And have fun."

"Watch those highway intersections," I smiled, replying back with our family's familiar phrase of warning.

She smiled at that, too. "I got you a calling card," she said, pulling a small piece of plastic from her purse and handing it to me. "Call us anytime, day or night. Okay?"

"Okay, I love you."

"I love *you*, Amelia Johnson. You know that? You can do anything you put your mind to."

We both choked up a bit at that. It was the same message she'd instilled in me my entire life, but it held so much more meaning now as I stood there on the precipice of my new one. A couple of tears slid down my cheek as we hugged. And a lump of emotion caught in my throat, preventing me from saying anything further. When just as we broke apart, I saw him in the distance—across the busy parking lot.

It was Marty.

We'd met only briefly once, earlier that spring, among a group of JJ's other university friends. Yet as he sauntered toward us, emanating more self-confidence than I'd ever managed to muster in my entire life, I realized he was even better looking than I'd remembered. I flushed, suddenly losing all awareness of the buildings, the park with its geese, or the bustle of students around me.

Marty was a few years older than I was. Tall, probably about six foot three, and buff—well-built and muscular. He was a man, and I became acutely aware in that moment that I'd only ever previously dated boys.

His jeans were torn, stylishly worn out, and perfectly low slung on his hips. While his T-shirt, one of those trendy surf brands like Rip Curl or Billabong, stretched taut across his strong biceps and chest.

I noticed it all.

His bright blue eyes were kind, and his smile was wide and welcoming, showing off his perfect teeth. I stood frozen as he neared, my eyes never straying from him as he ran his hand through his blonde, wavy surfer's hair, which he was wearing much too long. I found myself captivated by the act, wanting to run my own hands through it.

It was only as he took those last few steps toward us that it clicked he was here to help us move into our dorms. I wiped at my face and smoothed my hair on instinct, flustered and annoyed that JJ hadn't warned me of this in advance.

"Are we ready to go?" he greeted us all casually—still smiling, but his gaze didn't linger. It seemed kind that he was trying not to draw attention to the fact that my mom and I had both been crying. He simply picked up our luggage in one fell swoop and started to lead the way toward our building.

JJ fell easily into step beside him, chatting animatedly with a duffle slung over her shoulder and her ponytail swinging with each step. But my eyes remained focused on the back of Marty's broad shoulders, and my heart pounded as I watched his retreating frame.

Then, in silent awe, I followed him inside.

SICK

EIGHTEEN YEARS OLD

My first year didn't unfold how I'd always imagined it would.

I'd arrived at university only five months after Kristin's death, and in many ways, I still wasn't myself. I couldn't talk about her or even hear the word cancer. I avoided any movies, television shows, or books that could trigger emotion, especially despising Nicholas Sparks novels for that very reason. I felt raw and fragile, and I was afraid to feel anything at all. I just wanted to throw myself into the excitement of university. I wanted to move on.

Perhaps evidence of that mindset was that I broke up with Cole only a week into the school year. I'd always suspected that there was no long-term connection there, but that fact had become clear over the summer months. He'd annoyed me with his neediness and immaturity, attempting to hold me back when I suddenly desired to be free.

I'd outgrown a lot of things that summer, and my relationship with Cole wasn't any different. Moving out, becoming an adult, and starting university had only further exposed our differences, solidifying my decision. It was the right thing to do, even if it did further disrupt my sense of normalcy.

I was missing basketball. I'd been scouted to play for the best team in the country at the time—the University of Regina Cougars—but no matter how hard I'd tried with my training, I hadn't been able to recover from my knee injury and subsequent surgery in time for the season. It had destroyed my dream of ever playing for the Cougars, let alone the WNBA.

I lost a part of myself when I lost basketball.

It had been my identity for seven whole years, and starting a new school year without it felt unnatural. I was more lost without *it* than I was without Cole. I found I had to redefine myself—rediscover who I was and where I fit in the world, if I was no longer a basketball player. And along with all the other losses in my life at that time, I grieved the loss of my dream as well as that identity.

It wasn't the fun and excitement I'd been expecting for my first semester away.

I struggled with a flare of generalized anxiety and an upset stomach as I tried to adjust to all the new changes. I struggled to sleep at night, but then during the day, I fell hard asleep in massive lecture halls. Consumed by fatigue, I started to skip many of my morning classes altogether.

It was JJ who anchored me when everything else was slipping away. She was in her final year of university, and her dorm room was just down the hall from mine. She helped me get some meds, and we worked through my angst together, walking for hours every day along the river in Wascana Park. Step after step in the sunshine, this time spent with my sister was healing. The anxiety soon started to fade away and my eternal optimism began to shine through again. I was finally finding a rhythm in my new life, and a few weeks of that first semester went exactly as I'd always imagined: new friends, dorm shenanigans, junk food, and late nights at the library.

And then it all fell apart.

It all started on a Friday night, or maybe it was early in the wee Saturday hours when I woke to the sound of the fire alarm. My first thought was that it was a drill.

I stumbled out of bed and into my slippers, threw a coat over my pajamas, and padded outside to join everyone else. I assumed it wouldn't take very long.

The fire trucks were already arriving as I stepped outside to join the group huddled in the parking lot, standing underneath the glow of the nearest street light. It seemed odd to have a practice drill in the middle of the night, especially when the temperatures were well below freezing. And as we watched the men in uniform start to file out, I also found it odd that so many needed to come on-site just to turn off an alarm.

However, as the minutes continued to tick by, and we soon neared an hour of standing in the freezing cold with the firemen yet to return, it became apparent that this was not a drill. Rumors started to circle among the crowd that one of the girls had left a candle burning on the seventh floor.

We fidgeted impatiently as time continued to pass, with only those rumors and no actual explanation as to what had occurred. When finally, a fireman walked out the front doors and gave us a wave.

"All clear," he called. "You're good to go back inside now."

We were agitated by that point, exhausted and cold, and I charged ahead first—antsy to crawl back into my bed. But as soon as I entered the building, the fireman stopped me in my tracks.

"The elevator's out of service," he said. "You'll have to take the stairs."

I rolled my eyes and sighed deeply at him, mustering all the attitude I could for an eighteen-year-old in fuzzy-yellow duck slippers. Then I marched haughtily over to the steel door of the emergency stairs, turned the handle, and flung it open.

I flew backward as a wall of water rushed past me. I fumbled, gripping the door for balance, and stumbled into the person standing behind me. We were like a lineup of stunned human dominoes, each bumping into the next as a river of water cascaded past us.

Apparently, the sprinklers had gone off, but the firemen hadn't thought to warn us.

Water had filled the stairwell. Water gushed down over our ankles.

Water was everywhere. We all stood holding onto each other in stupefied silence, afraid to be knocked down by the force. We waited for what felt like a lifetime for the water to disperse, the waterfall to lessen, until it was only a few shallow inches that streamed down the stairs and over my soggy duck slippers.

We had been freezing cold, and now we were wet. Exhausted, angry, and anxious to get back upstairs to see what we would find, we climbed the concrete stairs. One floor after another, we trudged through the still-flowing waters.

When we reached the fourth floor, I braced myself this time, cautious as I opened the steel door that exited the stairwell. We froze in the hallway as a pack. Standing in several inches of water, we peered over each other's shoulders—eerily silent as we watched.

Personal possessions floated past us. Flip flops and slippers. Plastic bins filled with unknown items. Papers. So many papers.

"Open all the doors!" someone yelled.

"Unplug all the computers!" called another.

We all ran in opposite directions, trying to save everyone's belongings. We flung open every door, unplugged every computer, and heaved everything we could lift up off the floor and out of the water.

It wasn't until after a panicked hour of this, that I finally ran past JJ's room. Her door, like all the others, had been propped open, and I saw that she sat cross-legged on her bed, peacefully eating a small yogurt and reading. Chaos surrounded her, yet she sat there totally composed—a perfect example of the stoicism she'd inherited from our dad. And for the first time that night, I laughed out loud.

She wasn't wrong to sit there and read; the amount of damage was more than any of us could possibly resolve. In fact, by that point, there wasn't much else any of us could do except follow her lead. Lucky for us, on the fourth floor, the beds were still dry.

Morning came much too quickly, only a few hours later, and the emergency response teams moved in. They set up massive commercial fans to dry out what was salvageable and proceeded to rip out the rest: the drywall, carpets, and standard-issue dormitory furniture.

Every door was left open, and the sounds of the fans screamed away. But without any other place to relocate us, we all continued to live among the destruction.

A few weeks later, my health fell apart.

I came down with mononucleosis along with some type of inflammatory hepatitis. And I had no sooner recovered from any of those ailments when I contracted shingles. And then the mono came back again.

I started having unprovoked issues with my heart—episodes of tachycardia. Chunks of my long blonde hair fell out as my body became jaundiced. My eyes and skin turned a bright yellow, and my urine was the color of Coke.

I remember waking up confused to find my face flat on the cafeteria table—my sister and our friends had all been eating their dinners around me while I'd apparently slept next to mine.

I remember waking up cold and alone on the floor of my tiny bathroom. In a panic, I launched myself at the toilet to vomit violently, my stomach contents devoid of anything except bile and an antiemetic.

And I remember waking up in my bed to find that JJ was studying at my desk—her attempt to keep an eye on me—and her forcing me to drink some water. Yet when I tried to smile and thank her, I found that it was no longer JJ who sat there but Lana. And when I went to ask Lana where JJ was, it was suddenly Chantelle.

I was told that JJ eventually called my parents—as I awoke to find myself with my dad in his truck, already halfway home on the highway, headed back to Moose Jaw.

I remember lying prone on the sofa in my parents' basement.

And fainting, falling into the arms of the nurse at the hospital.

I remember all of those experiences as still images. Moments frozen in my mind. But the images remain disconnected from one another, with no recollection of anything having happened in between.

EXPLOSION

I could tell *it* was happening again.

I was on edge, and I could feel it building. I'd been mildly unsettled all day, bothered by a conversation I'd had on text with my friend Andrea just that morning. I felt misunderstood, and very disconnected.

It shouldn't have been a big deal, and logically, I did know that—but there was no part of me that was feeling logical that day. Vexed by a niggling anxiety yet unable to put my finger on exactly why, I wanted to try and talk it out with my husband, get past the angst.

I should have known it wouldn't be that easy.

I hadn't slept for so many nights in a row that I'd long lost track. With the pressure from the encephalitis and the resulting migraine, all on top of a jaw that kept screaming at me, I could barely see through the white-hot pain. Sitting there in our kitchen, I was barely holding on.

My tone came out too sharp as I snipped a quick response at him, and I cringed internally at both the resulting pain from trying to use my jaw, as well as how bitchy I'd sounded. I wasn't proud of it; I knew I'd been irritable, difficult to be around all day. The burden of what I'd been carrying was so obviously crushing me.

I wasn't mad at my husband—far from it.

I was tired.

The constant pain, the fear, the sensory overload, the day-to-day monotony of being chronically ill—I was *tired*. My snippy response had been the best I could manage. I didn't even have the energy or the mental capacity to utter another word, not even an apology, and I hated myself for it. All I could do was lay my head on our kitchen table and close my eyes, trying to forget it all.

My brain had been scrambling on and off all day. Short-circuiting. Like the image one sees when an old-fashioned television loses signal and goes to static—chaotic zigzags of light and dark. Moments where the fast-forward button had been pushed, and all my thoughts and emotions became an incomprehensible whirl. As if my mind had gone through the blender.

However, as I sat there, with my head on the table in front of me, the brain fog rolled in. Unhurried and unassuming. It was a stark contrast to the speed of the blender. Now everything was slowed down.

Way down.

I should have seen it coming. I should have taken precautions and hidden myself away, away from the fog and my unsuspecting husband.

But I didn't.

It engulfed me; permeating me, seeping into all the recesses of my mind. I was underwater, and everything had been weighted down, embogged like in a dream. I could still hear my husband's voice off in the distance, but now it was garbled. Was he checking on me? The words were so unexpectedly slow that I couldn't make any sense of them. Their usual cadence was gone, drowned under the heaviness of the fog.

I knew inside, intuitively somehow, that the issue had to be with me. It had to be my brain that had slowed—not the world nor his speech—it was me.

I was frustrated by that, but my immediate frustration only clouded my mind even further. I snapped again.

I was confused by the fog and my inability to understand and then embarrassed by my own confusion. I got defensive. Triggered by a fear that I was misunderstood and disconnected from those around me, stemming from an even greater fear that there was something wrong with me—my brain simply glitched.

I instantly felt everything too intensely. Everything in me was exacerbated; my nerves on fire.

I knew I had to shut it down. Ashamed of my attitude and tone of voice, I knew I had to stop it and stop it fast—before *it* had a chance to happen again. So in my attempt to put a halt to the fog, the glitch, and the blender, I shouted—but immediately knew that hadn't been the right call either.

The pain ripped through me as I ripped my jaw open—injuring myself. Yet even though I knew there would be a price to pay for that act, still, I was unable to quit.

Words burst out of me in a frantic attempt to stay in control, to quiet the chaos in my mind, and make it all stop. To explain myself. To express myself. To prove my point. But everything was so scrambled that I couldn't even remember what my point had been.

I didn't mean half of what I said. Although admittedly, I wasn't sure what I'd said. And I didn't get any time to work it out in my mind before I was abruptly thrown into playing a part; a scripted performance I was required to follow. The words, the actions were no longer even my own.

I watched myself from across the room—my other self—the woman who wasn't quite me. She was in the bedroom now, unsure how she'd even gotten there, and she was furious—though simultaneously trying not to laugh at the absurdity of it all. Unstable, yet through the madness of spinning thoughts and emotions, she tried desperately to appear normal. To remain poised, sound intelligent, and communicate effectively.

I was paradoxically both the lead actress and the audience watching myself perform.

I couldn't even see if the man was in the room with her; I just watched as the longer it went on, the more the woman bought into it. The more indignant she got. And I couldn't take my eyes off of her.

She was visibly distraught. She may not have known what she was arguing about, but she knew how she *felt*. And in that moment, she could only see and perceive through that fallible lens. Fury and fear, and heartache and confusion all piled up on one another. Drowning her. Consuming her so completely, it stole all sense of perspective and rational thought, and at its mercy, she followed the erratic emotions blindly.

She followed *my* erratic emotions blindly.

Despair. Grief. Sorrow. Rage.

I wanted to throw something, punch the wall or something, anything to break the spell—but that's never been my style. Instead, I lashed out with my words. I said the wrong things, I yelled the wrong things, and I became an absolute monster. Thoughts and words tumbled out of my broken jaw so quickly that they didn't make any sense. I was hysterical, anguished to communicate some deep, dark part of myself—some great truth. Even if I wasn't sure myself what that great truth might be.

I screamed, and I sobbed, and the man was maybe still there somewhere in the background—trying to help me, trying to understand. It wasn't about him though, and it never had been. Still I got the sense he was trying to follow along, trying to keep up. But there was no keeping up with me. I was a wild woman, a freight train that could not be stopped.

I was not upset.

I was out of control.

It was extreme dysregulation—cognitive, emotional, all of it. Any stimuli only further fed my fire. And I knew then, for the briefest of seconds, as everything around me completely faded away—the man, the room, everything—that *it* was about to happen.

There was no stopping *it* now; I was too far gone.

I exploded.

Like I was possessed.

Like there was something inside of me trying to get out.

I collapsed on the ground in a heap as a bloodcurdling scream erupted out of me. My frozen jaw wrenched open as far as it would go to allow the screams out—as if two invisible hands had unceremoniously grabbed ahold of me and torn it apart.

I'd disappeared. Disconnected, gone from reality. Yet my body still screamed from the depths of its soul—no words, just screams. High pitched and shrill. As it pounded its fists into the ground and frantically grasped at its head. Pulling at its hair. Kicking and thrashing. Pushing and pulling itself along the floor, ricocheting off furniture. It held the scream longer than anyone knew was possible.

Screaming. Still screaming.

My husband would later tell the Lyme-guy that I transformed instantly into a wild animal. That my body contorted violently, writhing like nothing he'd ever seen before. And that over and over, I howled a bone-chilling, high-pitched wail as if I must be dying.

I have only a minimal recollection of any of that.

I only know in the end, as I finally emerged from the psychosis, that I was devastated at the realization *it* had happened again. I was full of self-hatred, heartbroken, and remorseful as I sat curling my shoulders inward, wrapping my arms around my balled-up legs. I retreated into myself, trying to hide who I was and what I had done. My body rocked back and forth with my sobs, gut-wrenching, deep-hitching wails of shame coming straight from my heart.

I was surprised to discover that my husband was still there, staring at me in shock. And I wondered if he'd been there the entire time—if he had seen *it* happen.

My paranoia immediately interpreted his expression as judgment. He was surely repulsed by me. He feared me, despised me even. And for *it*, I was certain he was going to leave.

I had to make him understand that it wasn't my fault. I wanted to tell him it wasn't my fault. But I hesitated to say that aloud because I was starting to wonder if it was even true. I was afraid that through all this, I'd only ever proven his suspicions correct—that I really *was* crazy. And maybe *that* would be the next role I would be forced to play.

The dysregulation was starting all over again.

My brain glitched, and I winced, as if a phonograph needle had been pulled violently across the vinyl record that was that exact moment. I lost both visual and audio, with everything scrambling again and coming to a screeching halt. My brain short-circuited. My thoughts were thrown through the blender for a second time. A third.

The episodes started to roll one after another, picking up speed. One ended, and another began. I was lost and drowning in the glitches, questioning my perception of reality and unable to trust my own thoughts. I wanted to laugh out loud at the realization that I'd been keeping a secret.

I really *was* crazy.

And the fact that a crazy person lived inside of me was starting to scare me.

I obviously had no control over myself or what was happening; I was not even capable of coherent thought. I'd become but a victim, tied to the tracks, struggling and afraid as the runaway train that was my mind raced threateningly toward me.

My eyes widened as I scampered frantically back, wedging myself into the corner of the room. I was breathing heavily now and physically shaking, and as my husband saw this, he backed away, giving me the space I needed.

He had seen me do this before, too many times before. Still, I screamed at him to not touch me. Terrified, hyperventilating, I was unsafe in my surroundings.

No. Unsafe in my mind.

I detached again. Dissociated from my mind and my body, I tried to go somewhere safe. But just as I arrived there, to a foggy nothingness, another short circuit startled me alert. The emotions. The thoughts. The fears. Whirling through the blender again. A flood of adrenaline.

A panic attack.

The more he talked, the worse it got—I didn't even know what he was saying. He was talking; his lips were moving, but I couldn't hear anything.

I am deaf. I am DEAF! I screamed. Though the words didn't come out; they were only in my mind.

I didn't understand. I couldn't admit that I didn't understand—I would sound crazy! But I was not crazy. I could not. Be. Crazy.

Something was definitely wrong—what was wrong with me? WHY did this keep happening?

PANIC.

Racing, half-formed thoughts bombarded me again, tormented me, and clouded my ability to process thought. Clouded my ability to process anything at all. My brain was a jumbled mess of thoughts and emotions coming at me in rapid fire, convulsing in a seizure.

I stopped breathing.

My heart pounded, and as waves of heat washed over me, I was simultaneously freezing cold and sweating. Dizzy and disoriented. Shaking uncontrollably. My chest hurt, and I jammed my fingers into the intercostal spaces between my ribs overtop of my heart, trying to make the pain stop.

I couldn't breathe. I couldn't breathe. I COULDN'T BREATHE.

In an instant, I was floating above the room—watching myself again—my pained body rigid below.

I watched it sitting frozen.

Panicking. Deaf and mute.

My husband was still talking to it, completely unaware of the hearing loss. Unaware that I was no longer in that body, no longer even in that room.

I'd gone crazy.

I was absolutely crazy. And my body was going to die there if I didn't get its heart and breath under control.

The pain seared through me, and I wailed, rushing back into my body and throwing myself dramatically into the fetal position on the hard floor once again. I needed to stop. For my own self-preservation, I knew that I needed to stop. I could no longer exist in the pain of this moment. The threat was too high; the pain was sure to kill me. And a flash of lucidity washed over me as I realized I didn't want my husband to have to see this—to see me as crazy, even though I knew that I was.

My doctors had all tried to define the different stages of these episodes. An amygdala hijack. A total short circuit. Extreme dysregulation. Dissociation. Depersonalization. A limbic seizure. A panic attack. A psychotic break. And, of course, the theoretical "Lyme psychosis." But regardless of what name they all used, I just knew I needed help.

No one could do it for me.

I was going to have to save myself.

I pressed my hands into my ears and squeezed my elbows in toward each other, compressing my head as tightly as I could to block out the thoughts. Block out the pain. The fear. I sobbed uncontrollably, and I focused on that—focused on trying to get my breath back. Squeezing my head as hard as I could, I rocked back and forth, pressing my face into the corner of the wall. I crushed my skull between my hands. Then I gasped a final, deep, guttural breath—all too aware of the physical pain ripping through me. And mustering all of my strength and focus, I broke through the thick, heavy curtain of confusion that was suffocating me, the panic that was paralyzing me, and I screamed at the top of my lungs:

"GET OUT. GET OUT. GET OUT."

It's a half day later when I eventually rouse here—somehow, now in my bathroom—only to discover myself shattered all over the floor.

I can see the millions of pieces of me scattered around—broken, jagged, and fragile. An ugly mess of detritus dumped across our beautiful tile.

My gaze rests on each part, and I know I'll have to move on. I'm going to have to pick up those pieces, careful to not slice myself any further with their sharp edges. I will have to clean up the mess on the floor. The mess that is me.

I will have to piece all those shattered fragments together again—find a way to make them fit, make a presentable whole. A convincible whole. I'll have to secure them together somehow, some way, so that they cannot break apart again. I will have to secure them more tightly this time so that there will not *be* another next time.

There cannot be. Any more. Next times.

And finally, I will have to hide the ugly seams, hide my scars away from the world.

I have done this all before.

But I cannot yet muster up the energy, the strength, or the courage to begin again.

I am still frozen.

I am still shattered.

I will need to hide in the darkness, among the mess of myself, for a little while longer.

LOVE

NINETEEN YEARS OLD

Right from the very start, I knew there was something different about Marty. I found myself drawn to him without even really realizing it myself. My eyes scanned hallways automatically, my body wandered aimlessly through crowded parties—until finally, I found myself standing next to him.

It wasn't for his obvious good looks or even his charming sense of humor. It was how I *felt* whenever I was around him. A slight flutter in my heart and a catch in my breath. An ache, a pull, a need that could only be filled when he was near.

In a way, it was odd that he had that effect on me; we were new friends and didn't even know each other that well yet. But there was something about him, something about being in his presence—I didn't need to know everything to know that he felt right.

It was our timing that was always wrong.

My life as a university student was hectic once again, and it pulled me in different directions. I'd missed a lot of school when I was sick, but even once I was back for the winter semester, Marty and I had completely different schedules and groups of friends. And the locations of his classes were never anywhere near mine. We rarely ran into each other in the halls.

We were always crossing paths at the wrong times (like embarrassingly when I was with a boyfriend), and at the right times, Marty was nowhere to be found.

I'd dated Cole, and then there was Rob. I was getting asked out fairly often, and the boys I hung out with and the dates they took me on were always just fine. But I could never describe them as anything more than that. I rarely felt comfortable, and I certainly never discovered any deep connections. I didn't know if a part of me still wasn't ready for dating or if what I thought was lingering anxiety was actually intuition—my inner voice trying to tell me that I was with the wrong guy.

Either way, there were a lot of first dates and not a lot of seconds.

I spent my summer break back home in Moose Jaw, working again at the Owl Centre. I thought about Marty the entire time. I even tried to "accidentally" run into him after work one day when I'd heard he might be in town. I drove around most of the evening, keeping my eye out for gatherings at different venues—it wasn't exactly a well-thought-out plan, and it didn't prove successful. I didn't have any luck.

When I returned to school in the fall, I decided I was done with tiptoeing around; I was ready to put myself out there. However, as I stepped confidently on campus for my second year, I was shocked to discover that Marty had already moved to Calgary for an internship, and no one had thought to tell me.

I sat with this news for a few days, and then I sent him an email. I wanted to test the waters, see how he felt. I needed to know, needed an answer. But when weeks passed by without a response from him, I embarrassingly felt I'd gotten just that.

There wasn't much time to dwell on the rejection though, as I was quickly consumed by my second year of university. And with the exception of my dating life, things were exactly how I'd always imagined.

I'd changed majors and settled easily into my new psychology and sociology courses, soon reaching the top of my class. I was scouted for modeling, and I was even back to playing basketball—even if it was only recreationally.

I had a ton of friends and we loved dressing up to go out dancing and to parties. We skipped classes in lieu of random shopping trips, went on ice cream runs even when it was minus forty out, and we had decadent waffles with strawberries and whipped cream nearly every single weekend. I thought living in the university dorm surrounded by my friends was a blast.

Marty remained in the back of my mind, however, and so I declined when Liam asked me out for the first time. He was newly popular on campus and known for being funny; in fact, my friends were all obsessed with him. Though I wasn't sure I got the attraction.

It was when he asked me out a second time, and then a third, and I still hadn't heard anything from Marty, that I gave in. I figured if my friends all liked Liam that much, there must be something I was missing.

There wasn't. I learned the hard way that Liam wasn't the type of person I wanted to be around at all.

Liam hid behind his humor, while I found him crude. And I swiftly broke up with him one dramatic night after I'd refused to have sex with him when he'd pressured—not listening and nearly forcing.

It hadn't taken me long to realize that Liam was a jerk, but the fact that I'd spent any of my time with him at all had been tremendously *too* long. I felt dirty and gross.

I decided I was done with dating, not wanting to waste any more of my heart. It seemed I'd only been getting attention from bad boys who gave me anxiety, or boys I felt sorry for and dated to avoid hurting their feelings. And I knew neither was right.

In January, Marty returned to school and reentered my life.

We decided to go out for ice cream one night as a chance to catch up. He drove us to the local Dairy Queen, where we both got Blizzards, and we took them to eat in the warmth of his truck. All alone in the privacy of the vehicle, nibbling on our ice cream, we slowly, hesitantly revealed a bit more about our semesters apart.

"I emailed you," I said casually.

"You did? When?"

"Last semester, when I realized you weren't at school."

"Oh."

There was a brief pause while I analyzed his *Oh*. "I wondered why you didn't reply."

"I never got it!" His voice was suddenly filled with an enthusiasm I couldn't identify. Was it defensiveness? Excitement?

"Oh," I said weakly, staring at the ice cream in my hands. My brow furrowed as I took another spoonful.

"What did it say?" he prodded, not letting the silence drag on.

I knew I was stuck. The nervous energy was starting to build in my chest—I was the one who'd started this conversation, I couldn't get out of it now.

A part of me wanted to boldly tell him all the things I suspected I felt deep down but had never dared put into words. Not with friends, or JJ, or even in the privacy of my own room. Things like *I like you, I want you*, and *I think I always have*. Instead, I stammered a lot, my face flushing in the dimness of the cab as I struggled to find the right words.

"I... umm... I mean, and I thought maybe you..."

"I do," he cut in, somehow understanding what I'd been trying to say all along. And at his words, my face flushed scarlet once more.

"Well, I was confused when you didn't answer the email," I told him, a little braver, a little bit of attitude creeping back into my voice. But then I remembered my semester: the dates I'd gone on, the boys I had kissed, and my anxiety surrounding it all. I found myself wanting to confess it. Like if he could forgive me for my foolishness, maybe I could, too—and *we* could start anew. "I started dating Liam... and it was a mistake. A big mistake. I kissed somebody else when I was away. And I—I don't know what I'm doing." Tears filled my eyes.

"Well," he said kindly, saving me from my own anxious rambling. "When you're ready, if you want. I'm here."

Then we sat there, continuing to talk in the privacy of the vehicle long after our ice creams had been eaten and the other patrons had gone. Through the truck and store windows, we watched as the Dairy

Queen employees went about their closing routine: turning out the lights, locking the doors, getting into their own cars, and driving away, leaving us alone in the empty lot, still talking.

But now we weren't so nervous anymore. We started to share our thoughts and feelings more easily, and we laughed and laughed some more. All with our eyes locked in the darkness, the pale light from a single street lamp dimly illuminating the cab.

Our timing was finally right.

Our romance snowballed from there. A first kiss, a first date, and only a few months later, sitting on the tailgate of that exact same charcoal gray F-150 (this time in the middle of a wheat field), there was once again something big standing between us. Something that couldn't go on any longer; it had to be said.

It filled me so completely, building up a pressure in my chest and in the back of my throat—butterflies, I'd finally found my butterflies. They were overflowing me, escaping me, fluttering in my chest, and pulling on the corners of my mouth as I bit back my smile. And so in the light of mid-day without question or hesitation, insecurity or anxiety—for the first time in my life, not saying it to a boy as a polite response, but of my own accord—I stared into his eyes, his beautiful bright blue eyes, and definitively told him:

"I love you."

And it was fireworks.

Of all the rom-coms I'd watched and boy band lyrics I'd memorized, our real-life romance ended up superseding it all.

We were always holding tight onto one another's hands and grinning like fools. We talked for hours before bed each night, neither one of us ever wanting to hang up the phone. We were different, each with our own, unique interests and groups of friends, yet enough core similarities that our compatibility was easy. Our views aligned on all of the big topics.

He often surprised me with thoughtful gifts and handwritten letters. But he was there in the tough times, too, like when I had a flare in anxiety and struggled with anorexia as a result. Or when I came down with a strange flu and was unable to move due to shooting body pains; Marty had been the one I'd entrusted to physically carry me into the doctor's office, where they suspected I'd been infected with West Nile.

Behind his truck, he even once pulled a kite with a huge handmade banner attached, the words floating way up in the sky for everyone on campus to see.

I love you, Amelia.

At the end of that semester, I moved back home to Moose Jaw to work for my third summer at the Owl Centre, and Marty moved to Swift Current for another internship. I cried as our relationship was put to the long-distance test.

Weeks passed, and we wrote letters. We called every night and saw each other on weekends. We were doing everything we could to make it work. When two weeks before my twentieth birthday, I received a surprise delivery from the florist. A huge bouquet of flowers, pinks and purples, all arranged in a large glass vase. And a mysterious envelope arrived in the mail later that day.

Standing in the hallway of my childhood home, with my mother unable to contain herself from hovering over my shoulder, I opened the envelope—perplexed to find a very-pink, very-cartoony, Disney-princess-themed birthday party invitation. It was ridiculous.

I thought it must be some kind of mistake, so I turned it over to read the inscription:

Princess Amelia's Birthday Surprise
July 23rd
11:30 a.m.

I might have actually blushed.

I called Marty later that evening, knowing it could only be from him. And he confessed, admitting he'd had to buy the entire package of princess-themed invitations just to mail me that single one—though he refused to tell me anything more. A date and a time, but that was it. For the next two weeks my mom and I were left to wonder what he was planning, yet he never gave anything away.

When my birthday finally arrived, Marty picked me up at my parents' house promptly at eleven thirty. My family watched as he showered me with gifts, and then we headed off. I couldn't wait to get going. But Marty drove us straight to Crescent Park, which was only a five-minute drive from the house and not at all what I'd had in mind. A flash of uncertainty washed over me as he started to set out an elaborately romantic picnic for two *in Crescent Park.*

I felt very exposed there. It was a bit like that invitation he'd sent, cheesy, though I supposed it was heartwarming. It was a lot. The invitation, the weeks of suspense, my mother's excitement, the flowers, the gifts, and now a very public picnic? The practical side of me was feeling like maybe this was all over the top. Unnecessary. I stood there awkwardly as I watched Marty pull out items from the basket—I didn't know how to react. I felt a bit frozen in place.

It wasn't until I saw that he had perfectly cut up all of my favorite fruits and arranged them into tiny little containers for me that I eventually broke. It was those little pieces of fruit that ultimately got me—put me over the edge. And my heart burst at his effort and attention to detail as I sank onto the blanket beside him.

The grass was perfectly green, the sky a rich blue, and big oak trees arched high above us—but I just looked at *him.* And then, as it always was when we were together, my nerves immediately melted away.

The picnic was perfection.

"This will be the soundtrack for our secret road trip," Marty said, handing me a mixed CD once we were done eating.

I laughed, seeing that his eyes sparkled yet again with renewed mystery. "What do you mean? Where are we going?"

All he did was grin.

So we packed up the remains of our picnic and got back into his truck, where I settled in easily beside him. Our hands automatically intertwined, and I plugged in the new CD. New pop country music filled the cab, and we both started to sing along to the love songs as he drove us out of town. I found myself continually looking over at him—admiring his strong jawline, his right hand in mine, and the way his left hand rested casually on the steering wheel, the short-sleeves of his shirt riding up on his biceps a bit too tight.

I was the luckiest girl in the world.

We eventually ended up at Lake Diefenbaker, but oddly, I noticed we didn't turn down to the beach. Instead, he continued driving down empty country roads, occasionally missing a turn and having to backtrack. When just as it seemed like we were well and truly lost, he pulled the truck down a lane leading to a ranch.

I got out of the truck, confused and wondering if he'd stopped to ask for directions. As I looked around at the barns and farm animals and the house in the distance, I saw an older-looking cowboy was striding toward us.

"Happy Birthday," the man called out in a big, booming voice without missing a beat. With no further words or explanations, he simply stepped right up to me and thrust the reins of a horse into my hands.

I'd told Marty only once that riding was something that I loved, but living in the city never got to do. My heart swelled with the instant realization that he'd remembered that very brief comment and arranged this private excursion just for us.

Marty was like that. The gifts he gave and the dates he planned were always so *big*—full of romance and mystery and thoughtful little details. Yet as my mind went through all that he had done for me that day, and in recent months, I knew I didn't need any of it. I didn't need banners or flowers or picnics or princess-themed birthdays.

I only needed him.

Being with Marty felt right on all levels. I'd never made a list of characteristics that my perfect man would possess, never known what it was that I'd wanted or needed until I'd found it all in him.

He felt like home. And I think I'd always sensed it. Even before we'd begun dating, somehow I'd always known—and been in love with him all along.

I'd been in love with him right from the very start.

We spent the rest of that day and into the evening exploring the countryside on horseback. We chatted and laughed as we rode side by side, pointing out wildlife and the beauty of the lake off in the distance. We only stopped occasionally to reach for each other's hands or steal a kiss. Sometimes we even raced. Over the hills and through the valleys, we literally rode off into the sunset together—the prairie sky all around us alight in flaming shades of pink, orange, and gold.

It was our very own fairy tale.

BURDEN

I have eighty-nine symptoms. I'm in constant pain and misery, fainting every time I try to stand up—yet somehow, I still notice that my husband is cute.

Marty and I have been married for fifteen years now, and in some ways, he is still the boy I fell in love with; he is still tall and broad-shouldered, with that beautifully thick, dark blonde hair. But after so many years together, I know him better. I've amassed more data. So, I can confidently say that he's *not* the same guy he was when we started dating in 2003.

He's better.

He was always smart, but he's only gotten more so with age, and I'm proud to say that I've watched him parlay that into a very successful career. He's grown into a leader, both at work and with friends and family. He's well respected and admired, the guy everyone calls for advice. Yet he has always remained incredibly humble, genuinely happy to help, both kind and generous with his time. And he's fun. The first person to jump cannonball style into a pool or dive headfirst off the boat. He makes everyone around him feel comfortable with his self-deprecating humor and his playful, warm, and welcoming nature.

He's laid-back, doesn't stress, and can remain calm in absolutely any situation. I am in awe of him. And he's been an amazing partner to me all of this time, always treating me with kindness and respect and providing unwavering support. He's been the yang to my yin. He's been my rock.

He's stood with me through fear and through pain, listened to every single crazy symptom, and researched right alongside me. He's driven me to every test, every blood draw, and sat through endless appointments speaking for me. I've really had to lean on Marty, even literally, to get out of chairs, out of bed, hobble across the house, or into those appointments.

He's done it all alone. He has supported me no matter how much of a disaster I've been—how unstable or unreasonable. He has stayed.

And if I'm being totally honest with myself, he probably shouldn't have. It's not been fair to him. I know we can't continue on like this, ignoring the burden that I've become or the toll this mystery disease has taken on our marriage.

It might be me instead who will have to go.

I cried in front of the Lyme-guy yesterday. I didn't mean to; I may be completely running out of hope and giving up, but I was still confident that once I got into his office, I'd be able to push through my emotions and have the meeting. I am a pleaser, after all; I always act socially appropriate. Yet as I shuffled into his office for our February appointment, holding onto both Marty and my cane, I took one look at the Lyme-guy and broke down crying. Surprising even myself.

My beautiful Marty spoke for me then.

"The treatments continue to make her worse. She's in constant pain. Her jaw and her teeth are so painful that she's barely spoken or eaten in the last year and a half. She has a debilitating migraine every single day, continues to be electrocuted, and is suffering from a profound depression." He said it all so matter-of-factly, digging deep to convey what he knew needed to be said in the moment, somehow, without letting his own emotions about it get in the way. "She's giving up."

A deafening silence ensued.

How do you proceed with an appointment that starts like that?

My tears continued to fall, yet my body somehow fell into our regular routine. I simply took my seat in the familiar brown leather chair opposite the Lyme-guy's desk, and I handed him my notes. And then I stayed silent for him to read those notes aloud, as he always did. I knew my very first question at the top of page one was about to ask something difficult. It was a question my husband and I were both too afraid to voice out loud.

Is there someplace that would be willing to take me? A hospital or a clinic somewhere?

The Lyme-guy looked up from the page, met my eye, and compassionately shook his head no. There wasn't.

It had taken a lot for me in that moment to hand over the page of symptoms and questions that so very clearly exposed the severity of our situation. With him in his business attire, behind a double-pedestal desk—and me, embarrassingly with my cane and my shabby clothes. White socks with Birkenstocks because I couldn't even get proper shoes on my feet. And athletic wear (and not the nice stuff), with the straps of an old ratty swim top in lieu of an actual bra showing at my neckline. I felt pathetic in comparison, admitting I couldn't handle his treatment. Not only was it not helping me, I was still getting worse.

I'd always tried to stick to the facts with him, never wanting to waste any one of my precious forty minutes attempting to manage something so futile as my emotions—but I was desperate. And I suppose, in a way, that was a fact. The facade of stoicism that I usually wore to his clinic was obviously cracking.

"There is a clinic in Florida that, for $60,000, will treat you for six weeks," he said ruefully. "Although, unfortunately, they won't do anything different from my protocol here."

I gave a small nod of understanding, even though it wasn't what I had in mind. I knew I needed more than that. More than six weeks, and ideally full medical support. I needed a diagnosis I could have confidence in. And, if not a cure, at the very least, I would need something to offset some of these symptoms.

I'd seen it firsthand with friends suffering through cancer treatments. Certain side effects and symptoms were somewhat anticipated, so corresponding medications were provided in advance to alleviate them. But with this theoretical Lyme and its treatment, the Lyme-guy has only ever nodded his head and then sent me home to "handle it" alone—with not a single medication to offset any one of my symptoms. I haven't been offered a wheelchair because I can't walk or oxygen because I can't breathe. And I feel like we have to be missing something here. Surely, this can't be it. It doesn't even make sense that we've been left to solve this all on our own, now "handling" eighty-nine symptoms.

I need help. And it certainly isn't fair to Marty to be responsible for me in this way.

"Let's test you," the Lyme-guy said, interrupting my ruminations as he stood up and moved toward the exam table.

I was crushed as I numbly followed him—stabilizing myself by gripping the chair backs as I went, going through the motions of getting myself to his table and lying down, all without bothering to respond a single word. What was there to say? I just turned my focus, as always, to the dingy ceiling tiles above me, and I zoned out.

Too emotionally spent, too physically spent, I lay there with tears leaking out the corners of my eyes and running down through my hairline onto the Lyme-guy's table for the entire twenty minutes. And when the exam was over, I made my way back to the desk where the Lyme-guy "confirmed" that the infection was still active in my chest, my jaw, and my brain. Then he handed me a script for twelve new prescriptions and, with it, a feeling of utter hopelessness.

I'm worried he's going to give up on me. As each month that the Lyme-guy continues to reiterate that my case is tricky and my infection quite bad, we keep questioning his methods—telling him that he's only making me worse. And we don't have another plan B. There's been no progress, and we have no other theories. I'd actually love to leave the Lyme-guy myself, but we haven't found any other clinic willing to take me.

I guess I'm just supposed to be grateful for the Lyme-guy—that there is at least one doctor still willing to make an attempt at figuring out what's wrong with me. One doctor willing to risk his own career and reputation by prescribing against those guidelines. Even if the only support I get are wishes of good luck to handle the onslaught of pain that is sure to follow.

And I am grateful.

I am.

I'm just not sure I can do it anymore.

I never imagined this. When I said those vows at twenty-two years old, "in sickness and in health," I never imagined what a drastic turn life could take. Yet here we are.

I'm easily triggered and overreactive—unhappy, afraid, and in pain—and I project that all onto my poor Marty. He tiptoes around me at the house, as if I'm a crazy person. And he's probably right. With every single one of our "arguments" now my own doing, he's not even an active participant; rather, just a witness to my constant mental breakdowns.

We try to spend as much of our time apart in an attempt to avoid this conflict—or worse yet, one of my full-blown explosions. He often has to take himself outside for a walk, gone for two to three hours at a time, he just wanders the city sidewalks alone. Then, upon his return, he retreats immediately to the basement where he stays busy in the home office, exercises in the gym, watches TV, and now even sleeps in the guest room. I can see on his face the relief that this provides—it just hurts that I'm too unwell to go down there to visit him, even if, on some level, I do understand.

I'm afraid I've broken him. Broken us. He used to be open with his thoughts and feelings, but now, with the continual risk of triggering my new fragile state, he's had to close off and keep to himself. It's heartbreaking—to be so emotionally segregated as well as physically now, too.

We have no romance anymore, no emotional or physical closeness. No intimacy. And I miss the comfort of my husband; we used to hold hands and fall asleep every night intertwined. But now, I can't be touched at all, and that's a level of isolation most can't even imagine.

It's been seventeen months since anyone last hugged or held me for fear of triggering the electrocutions in my chest. I cannot be kissed for similar reasons (the electrocutions in my face and the fear of breaking my teeth with a misaligned jaw). And so obviously, if I can't be touched, there is no sex, and I miss the intimacy and connection of all those things. So much so that it's started to seep into my psyche.

I fear all he can see when he looks at me now are my crooked jaw, my pains, and my explosions. I am no more than a patient, a responsibility, and a burden. I know I am no longer a desirable woman. At the end of each day, when he pokes his head into my bedroom to say "goodnight" and "I love you," I hear his words for exactly what they are —mechanical. And so as I listen to his retreating footsteps, as he makes his way down to sleep in his basement, my eyes immediately start to well. I can simply no longer believe him.

I've spent an inordinate amount of time this last year researching conditions like bipolar, bipolar II, borderline personality disorder, and autism, trying to figure out what's wrong with me. At times, I've been convinced I have each of them—though, at other times, I'm convinced I have none. I've even asked my therapist Dr. Cathy, but yet again, as it was with the onset of my physical ailments, she became just another doctor in a long line of doctors to tell me I was "fine."

I don't feel right for this world.

The root of it seems to be a type of anxiety or panic attack that escalates into psychosis. Though I have heard some people in the medical community use the term "Lyme rage," I am not angry at anyone— except for maybe myself.

I scream to quiet the chaos that exists in my own head.

It is a projection of my pain; it is the voice of my fear.

It's an implosion of turmoil that's constantly tearing through me. Consuming me. Breaking me. Heartache and guilt and shame all tied up together in a knot that I can never unfurl.

It is more than I can bear.

So in the aftermath of yesterday's unsuccessful appointment with the Lyme-guy, I forced myself to crawl and stumble the fifteen steps from my bed to my desk, determined to research mental hospitals. My goal is to find someplace that will take me, seeing as no other regular hospitals will.

I fantasize about a place where my crazy won't seem so crazy, and a professional nurse can care for me. Medicate me. Sedate me even.

I've been sitting here for hours already this morning, since long before the sun will even think to rise. I'm wrapped in a blanket in the near dark, under the faint glow of a small desk lamp. I'm in the same ratty sweatpants and hoodie (now with inexplicable holes in the elbows), a heating pad on my ribs, and another tied around my jaw. As tears and snot continually leak down my face, a pile of used tissues sits on the corner of my desk in front of me, which I can see has now overflowed onto the floor.

I'm a mess. I research, I write, and I sob—they seem to be the only things I can manage. But I realized this morning that even a mental hospital would only be a temporary fix. They wouldn't be able to cure this mystery illness or fix my marriage. And seeing as I'm not in any type of true psychiatric emergency, it would be unfair of me to occupy resources that someone else might genuinely need.

Instead, I've moved on to researching real estate. I'm going to need someplace to live after the divorce.

It is I who always brings this up. I'm paranoid, convinced that *he* is going to leave *me*, so I make sure to say it first to give myself a false sense of control. Although I do also bring it up out of love—as an escape, a chance for him to save himself from me. I wouldn't even blame him if he took the out. I don't expect him to stay or love me like this; I don't see how he possibly could.

Divorce feels inevitable, even if it's not what I want.

I'm afraid to be out on my own, especially in this state. I'm unsure how to start over, and I'm completely at a loss as to where I would live. The Canadian border is still closed; the pandemic, no doubt, adds a level of difficulty to our situation. Even if, at the same time, I am oddly grateful for those closed borders.

I know I can't be around anyone. It's bad enough that I've been using JJ as my personal therapist—burdening her with my issues via text because it's more effective than talking to my actual therapist. But I can't have my family here in person. I need to protect them. I can't risk ruining the few relationships I have left.

I wouldn't be able to handle it.

I've grown to hate myself for this disease and those explosions. I despise what I have said and how I have behaved. I am haunted by who I have become. And though I might like to, I can't hate a theoretical Lyme or other disease for any of it. The explosions were mine and mine alone. I am the one to blame.

I've become a monster. An unhinged, messed-up disaster. And for that, I know these feelings are warranted, deserved even, so I don't allow myself to let go of my shame. As if possessed, I hold onto it as my punishment—convinced I don't even deserve to be forgiven.

I only dream of someday escaping it all.

I imagine curating perfectly communicated letters to each of my loved ones, explaining my situation and expressing my love. Then I would drift off to live somewhere on my own, somewhere I would not be a burden anymore, and this illness could not hurt anyone else.

The issue is that I am weak.

I hate that I'm hurting my family, and I hate that I'm not better for them—but selfishly, I still need them. Even if logically, I know I should run away. I should divorce my husband. Out of love, I should let them all move on with their lives and release them from the burden that I am.

But it is that same love, that makes it so impossibly hard for me to do.

NEW YORK

TWENTY-FIVE YEARS OLD

"It's in New York," Marty said while sitting on our bed, the TV on in the background, as he casually referenced the new job he'd been offered earlier that day. But that was as far as he was able to get before I burst out crying.

Looking around at our home, the hardwood floors, the vaulted ceilings, the palette of warm neutrals, I was proud of it. Proud of the life and the home we'd been building. We'd been happily married for three years at that point—married young, only a few months after my twenty-second birthday. And even though people had warned us that the first few years would be the hardest, we'd loved every minute.

Perfectly matched and probably annoyingly cute to those around us, we'd been falling more in love with each other every single day. Excited to experience all of our adult-firsts together, we'd started our careers and bought a house, and we'd been having a blast stumbling through buying our first pieces of furniture, painting the walls, and landscaping our new backyard.

We'd even adopted our baby, Pete—a loving and happy purebred American Cocker Spaniel. He had the silkiest soft fur, creamy vanilla white with beige, big feet that smelled like Tostitos, and comically large droopy ears. Though what I'd first noticed about him were his beautiful, trusting, and soulful green eyes.

He was perfect.

Our lives were perfect.

Pete was lying on the bed between us in that moment, and I absentmindedly ran my hand over his fur as I considered Marty's news. Living in northern Alberta, we were an easy five-hour drive for weekend visits with our families. We both enjoyed our jobs up in Lloyd, had a ton of new friends, and played on several recreational sports teams. Our life really was perfect; we couldn't have been happier. Full of hopes and excited dreams for our future, we were even both up for promotions at the time.

I was hoping to get a $15,000 raise, which I was quite proud of. I knew it wouldn't transform our lives, but it would be another step in the right direction. We'd had a scare the previous month when our dishwasher stopped working and been at a loss as to how we'd afford to repair it. My raise was going to give us a small, though very much-needed, cushion each month.

So why would we even discuss something so preposterous? Something so wild, like moving to another country?

I'd never dreamed of ever moving away. I enjoyed traveling, seeing the different cultures and landscapes and dabbling in different languages, but moving somewhere permanently was something entirely different. Something that had never even crossed my mind.

Canada was beautiful. It was safe and comfortable, and I enjoyed my life there. There wasn't anything I wanted to escape, not even the cold winters. And there wasn't anything I felt I was missing out on, anything else I needed. My life felt fulfilling just as it was—the three of us cuddled up together on our bed, watching an old rerun of CSI, with Canada as our home.

I hesitated to say any of that aloud, as my thoughts were still whirring in my mind. My immediate tears had shocked me, but not nearly as much as the news of his potential promotion. The raise he had been offered was more than ten times greater than the one I was expecting—yet we would have to move for it. And I didn't know how to feel about that.

It was obviously a massive opportunity, but in taking it, we would be choosing only one of our careers to pursue fully. The other person would have to play a supporting role. I would have to play a supporting role. I wouldn't even have to work in New York unless I wanted to. I could work solely for the personal satisfaction of it, without any of the financial obligation—and maybe that part did sound a bit appealing.

But again—the caveat—for this, we would have to move.

I ended up not responding at all; my heart and my mind obviously needed a chance to catch up. Neither of us had ever been to the northeastern states before, and I had no idea where the city of Horseheads even was. So I snuggled into Marty, burying myself deeper into the new feather duvet, as we continued to watch television in silence. An unspoken agreement had passed between us that we would table the discussion for another day.

And shockingly, I slept well that night, not giving New York a second thought. Yet, as soon as I awoke, it all came rushing back to me. I rolled over to shake Marty awake.

"Okay," I said, leaning over him, my long blonde hair spilling down onto the pillow and a bit over his face. Surprising even myself as a grin crept across my features with the excitement of an adventure that had already started to take shape in my mind. "Let's do it."

Marty's company acted quickly at the news of our agreement—quicker than either of us expected. They flew us out to New York the following week.

It was a whirlwind of a trip—full of excitement and a bit of anxiety. "Small" coffees the size of Big Gulps. Meals so large we ordered just one to share. "Small" towns with massive interstates running through them. And tours of "small" family homes at least twice the size of ours in Canada. Everything was bigger across the border.

On the last of our three days there, we made our choice and eagerly signed a purchase offer on a house still under construction (touring the framed structure and picking out finishes, all in one shot). Then we flew back to Canada to complete the final preparations: selling our home in Lloyd, applying for work visas, scheduling movers, and filling out piles and piles of paperwork to import our vehicles, our possessions, and even our dog. The weeks passed by in a blur.

I cried on our final night when saying goodbye to my new best friend Ang—she was soulmate material, and it felt way too soon to move away from her, only in the first few years of what should've been a lifelong friendship. And I cried again the next day when we drove through Moose Jaw, even though I knew my parents would be visiting us in a few short months. Then, just like that, less than eight weeks since we'd first even heard of a town named Horseheads, it was time to head for the border.

We were nervous about crossing; this would be our first time doing so, not as travelers but as an official relocation. We worried that the guards would have some issue with our paperwork or, worse yet, force us to quarantine our Petey. But we sailed easily through in less than an hour—our thick file of documents having checked out and the guards not giving the dog a second glance.

We crossed North Dakota and Minnesota, stopping briefly at the Mall of America to devour a huge American Cinnabon. We cruised through Wisconsin and Illinois, discovering for ourselves that Chicago really was quite windy. And finally, the homestretch through Indiana, Ohio, and Pennsylvania until we eventually crossed into the state of New York.

I glanced into the back of the SUV and smiled to myself, relieved Pete had settled in during the ride. I'd given him free rein in the car—folding down the seats in the back so that he could come and go as pleased, with easy access to his bed and a bowl of fresh water.

Yet he hadn't used any of it. Despite my efforts, he always chose to sit up front and sleep on my lap instead. We'd driven 3,425 kilometers over the span of three days, and for that entire time, Pete had lain across my lap. His little body, curled up in a ball like a fox, fit perfectly in the center of the nook of my criss-crossed legs, preventing me from moving at all.

But I liked it.

I turned away from the empty backseat and looked down at him in my lap, knowing neither one of us would have had it any other way. And I stroked Pete's silky vanilla fur while Marty and I talked and dreamed, making plans for what we wanted to see and do once we were settled. We'd only agreed to a short-term assignment in the States, and we wanted to hit the ground running—experience as much as we could and book flights for our families, too, so that we could all share in the excitement together.

Buzzed and overtired, we laughed as the hours passed, finding everything progressively a little bit funnier. Our bodies may have been stiff and sore, but our spirits were high as we drove those final hundred miles toward our new town.

I felt at home there—sitting in the car beside Marty, with Pete on my lap—even if we were technically homeless, in between places at that time. But home for me in that moment was less about being in a specific location and more about who I was specifically with. The important part was that we were embarking on this adventure together.

Stiff legs or not, I wouldn't have traded that feeling for anything.

PITTSBURGH

TWENTY-SEVEN YEARS OLD

Moving to America surprised me. The differences between countries were subtle, but they were everywhere. In many ways, it was a different world.

The New York accent was twangy and hard to understand at times, while as Canadians, we used British words yet spoke with our midwestern accents. The Americans laughed whenever we used the phrase "out and about," though they were confused if we spoke of double-doubles, toboggans, cutlery, or bunny hugs. It was all English, yet sometimes we couldn't understand each other.

At the grocery store, the products were all completely different (even the name-brand products I used to buy in Canada). As a result, those first few trips took twice as long as they probably should have. Meat didn't taste the same, but maybe that made sense, because nothing really tasted the same. And while we were used to government-controlled liquor sales from our time in Saskatchewan, in New York, the gas stations sold individual ice-cold beers at the checkout counter for you to take on the road.

The climate was extreme—the cold colder and the hot hotter due to the intense humidity. The rain fell harder, and the snow fell deeper, and we didn't have the right clothing for any of it.

It was all a little bit overwhelming, even the American people. It's not that they weren't nice; in fact, they were incredibly so. But they seemed to not have any boundaries, and we found them to be loud.

Much more outgoing and direct compared to their Canadian counterparts, the American people made intense eye contact when we passed them in the street and asked personal questions while we waited in line at the store. At house parties, new friends often broached topics that we found to be taboo—like openly asking about the details of our finances. We found it shocking, intrusive, and inappropriate, especially when strangers made small talk in the waiting room at the doctor's office, asked what I was in for, and then moved closer to tell me about their rash.

It was that same cultural friendliness that disturbed me in the waiting room, however, that made us feel included in New York. People rang our doorbell and welcomed us into the community with home-baked pies, cookies, and bottles of wine. Neighbors gathered on the street chatting animatedly after work (they didn't drive straight into their garage and put the door down immediately behind them like we'd seen them do in Alberta). And throughout the summer on our street, there was even an ice cream social every Sunday where each neighbor took a turn to host.

So these little differences certainly weren't all bad; they were just different. It was the bigger things I found harder to ignore. The culture shock was unexpected, it took some time for us to adjust to that.

I hadn't realized how accustomed I'd been to living in a country that leaned so far left, until I'd found myself in one that was falling off the spectrum to the right. Canada was a country with much more government control and a social safety net—a socialist influence. We noticed right away that it wasn't the same in the States.

The culture was different. The social systems were different. As an outsider looking in, I struggled to understand the nuances of the government or the political and health care systems. I felt like I was doing something black-market illegal the first time I had to pay a copay at the doctor's office, and I was saddened to see the greater division of wealth that existed south of the border. It didn't seem right, the dramatic contrast between the haves and the have-nots.

I didn't quite belong in New York. Even though I loved the adventure of it all, I always knew that I was just a visitor. It was a bit like being on an extended vacation (because, in a way, we were). We didn't know how long our placement in the States would be, so we embraced that vacation aspect every single weekend.

We traveled into New York City just to be a part of the action. We frequented different musicals and comedy shows and tried all the restaurants, loving the old architecture and the energy of the people. We hailed cabs, rode the subway, and even ate hot dogs from street vendors in Central Park. We were quickly becoming real New Yorkers. We didn't need maps, and we were constantly hosting friends and family from back home. We were so busy having fun we didn't even have time to miss Canada.

We went for scenic drives through the vineyards upstate, visited the finger lakes, and hiked with Petey in the forest among all the waterfalls. We'd been previously unaware that New York State even had so many.

My favorite of all was Watkins Glen. I found it surreal every time I journeyed inside that gorge where shale rock walls striated in different colors towered beside us as we went, moss and mushrooms growing within their cracks. The main trail took us past a whopping total of *nineteen* different waterfalls. At one point, the trail even passed behind a cascade where we could stand in the cool mist, smelling the wet rocks and peering through the falling waters at the vista of the deciduous forest beyond the gulch. It was a dream—especially in autumn, when the entire forest changed to red and gold. At every turn, there was a photo opportunity greater than the last.

The weekdays were a little less exciting, however. We'd made friends easily enough with two other expat couples from Western Canada. But with most everyone I knew busy with work, I found myself alone a lot. It was proving more difficult than either of us had anticipated for me to obtain a work visa and restart my career.

I spent most of my time making our new house into a home. It was a big colonial two-story with slate blue siding, black shutters, and white columns, and I immersed myself in the decorating and landscaping of it. I painted the odd accent wall and hung drapes. I spent weeks outside alone, building a picket fence for Pete and planting shrubs and perennials, including hundreds of tulip bulbs in anticipation of the next spring. And as I waited for the arrival of my work visa, I let my mind wander during these tasks, thinking about what it was that I wanted to do with my own career.

Thanks to Marty's promotion, we didn't technically need my income—he'd even suggested again that I take the year off. Yet I barely considered it. There wasn't any obvious reason not to work (we'd decided to wait on having kids until we returned home to Canada). But for me, it was bigger than that.

There was a *draw* to work. I was driven, just as I had always been growing up. Working hard and succeeding were integral parts of who I was; our new financial status didn't change any of that. I'd always enjoyed work, being part of a community, having my own work friends, goals, and successes. I found satisfaction, purpose, and value in that. And design had always been one of my passions; it even said so under my eighth-grade yearbook photo.

Future Career: Interior Designer.

So when my visa came through and an opportunity presented itself to work as a lead interior designer at the local firm downtown, I jumped on it.

Julie was my first New York client. Recently divorced, she told me she was afraid to live alone, afraid of being solely responsible for her daughter for the first time. Things were tense in that household, emotions ran high with the teenager angry in the aftermath of her parents' split. Julie was unsure of how to talk to her, how to navigate all of their combined feelings, let alone how to make their new house into a home. They were stuck emotionally, as well as physically, when I met them—their possessions a material representation of that stagnancy, all still untouched in their boxes months after they'd moved in.

I appreciated her willingness to open up to me. I recognized it might be scary to be vulnerable like that (even if it was an essential part of the design process). In the months I worked with Julie, that honesty allowed us to go much deeper than simple aesthetics. I helped her feel comfortable and safe in her new home. I empowered her to feel confident and proud, and I liked to think I even helped her find a bit of joy. I was passionate about design and architecture, but it was that ability to help someone transform their home, and sometimes even their life, that I found I loved the most.

I loved it so much, in fact, that I was starting to think about what it would take to start my own business.

I was hooked on design yet wary of the dishonesty I'd been seeing in the industry—horrified to witness other New York designers take advantage of their clients' vulnerability, gossip about entrusted information, and gouge those who obviously had money. I often thought of Julie long after her project had wrapped up and how important it was that the "Julies" of the world be properly taken care of.

But it was then, after only fourteen months of living in New York, that we got the news.

It seemed I'd only just set up our new home, secured a doctor and a dentist and somewhere for haircuts, and acclimated to the American way of life. We were only just starting to build our lives and careers in New York, finally planning for our future, when we heard Marty's employer was establishing a new head office.

And we were being transferred.

We were being transferred to *Pittsburgh*, and my mind instantly conjured a black-and-white image. Pittsburgh, in the early 1900s, a city that was devoid of color, devoid of life. A steel city with smokestacks that reached high up into a smog-filled sky, ash and soot covering everything in sight—including its people.

It's not that I was opposed to moving. New York, as lovely as it was, was only ever supposed to be a temporary assignment. I understood that.

Moving was fine. Expected. Exciting even.

But moving to Pittsburgh? I wasn't so sure.

I hardly had any time to process it at all. The weeks leading up to our transfer again passed in a blur.

My Grandma Smolinski unexpectedly died, and I flew back to Moose Jaw to be with my mom. Then it was just as I rushed back to New York to wrap up work, put the blue house for sale, look online for new digs, and organize movers, when my Grandma Johnson unexpectedly passed, too.

There wasn't any time for me to breathe, let alone think. And heartbroken, I didn't even have time to attend that second funeral.

Moving day was upon us in the blink of an eye. When finally, driving into Pittsburgh—Marty at the wheel and my Petey again on my lap—for the first time, the angst of the previous weeks started to fade away, and an excitement washed over me. I realized how dated my initial thoughts had been.

Pittsburgh was vibrant.

Situated at the confluence of three rivers, Steel City had blossomed into the City of Bridges—four hundred and forty-six in total, to be precise—bright, happy yellow arches over blue waters with little white boats meandering below. Lush green parks trailed the rivers, and skyscrapers filled the downtown—their pristine, shiny glass reflecting the deep blues of a perfectly clear sky. Two inclined railways with bright red cars transported tourists up the treed hillside. People casually ate at outdoor cafés, and giggling children ran barefoot through fountains.

This city was alive, colorful, and joyous.

It wasn't long before more Canadian expats transferred down to join us in Pittsburgh later that summer. We were all away from home and separated from our families, and we bonded in that, becoming each other's support systems. And our small group of three couples doubled in size.

We enthusiastically explored the city of Pittsburgh together, regularly attending professional football, hockey, and baseball games. We boated and jet-skied on the many rivers and lakes, celebrated all the holidays and birthdays together, and spent long weekends away exploring the surrounding sights in Ohio, Maryland, Delaware, DC, and even the Carolinas.

It was a good life, yet I sensed the two quick relocations were catching up to me. For as beautiful and fun as Pittsburgh was, my initial excitement for an adventure in the States had started to fade. A feeling of unsettledness was creeping in.

The company had rented a home for us this time (which was a relief not having to buy), but it was six thousand square feet of not-at-all-my-style. Yellow walls, with yellow drapes puddling on golden yellow traditional oak floors. Unnecessary moldings and columns throughout. Arches galore, hexagonal-shaped rooms, and tray ceilings in odd, not-quite-oval, not-quite-rectangular shapes. On top of it all, it had a floor plan that didn't make any sense—three stories, with a detached garage outside of the basement, and a driveway so short and steep it wasn't even useable.

I knew I had nothing to complain about, but architecture and design meant a lot to me and had always directly impacted my comfort in any given space. And we weren't allowed to make any changes to the rental or even install a fence for Pete, so the yellow house never did feel like it could be our home.

Compounding that feeling, we didn't have many visitors, as the name Pittsburgh didn't resonate with most of our friends and family from back home either. The months stretched on endlessly, until we had to acknowledge our reality. We were alone in the States, two thousand miles away from our families, and no amount of new friends or adventure could compensate for that.

I was suddenly aware of how different my life was—noticing for the first time that my sister and our other friends back home seemed so comfortable, having built their lives in only one location. Whereas, with our continual relocations, our sense of community was really quite small.

I was an outsider. First in Lloyd, then New York, and now in Pittsburgh. I blindly followed GPS directions, never entirely sure where I was or where I was going. I was forever the new girl, always having to find a new doctor, dentist, hair stylist, and gym. And I was tired of having to stop and restart my career.

We'd been away long enough that even Canada didn't feel the same. And compared to the seeming comfort and simple ease of my friends' lives back home, I had a looming sense that while I could fit in everywhere, I now belonged nowhere.

I tried to ignore this discomfort and instead threw my energy into furthering my education with online courses in interior design. Diving into my studies and learning insatiably, I dedicated my days to achieving my certifications. I met with a lawyer to file for my business license and took control of my career, officially starting my own company: AJ Design.

I hired a professional photographer and a website designer. I built an online presence, acquired all of the latest and greatest design software, and I hit the streets to establish trade relationships. I really dove right in. I took on jobs of all sizes, from decor and home staging to complete renovations and new construction. My projects ranged anywhere from a few hundred dollars to a couple million, simply because I liked helping people. And I stood behind my beliefs to treat my clients' money like it was my own, not only respecting but embracing the challenge of delivering big design on any budget.

My name started traveling in circles like wildfire—my clients, I guess, were impressed. I never had to advertise even once to stay busy. It was exactly what I'd always wanted.

It was my health, unfortunately, that got in the way, causing me to hit pause when I'd only just begun. There was something I'd been ignoring. Something I couldn't ignore any longer.

I'd had some digestive issues over the years—ever since that first year of university, actually—but the progression of my anxiety since moving to the States had only made those issues worse. And the worse my stomach got, the more anxiety it gave me. Yet the more anxiety I had, the worse my stomach got. I'd become trapped in a vicious and embarrassing cycle, and the last thing I wanted to talk about was anxiety, let alone my digestion.

All I wanted was to keep progressing in life and in my new career; but in my attempt to avoid what I was going through, the power my anxiety had over me only grew. And somehow, my relatively minor generalized anxiety became an all-consuming terror.

I spent the next few months making up excuses.

"Hi, yes, this is Amelia Johnson calling. I need to cancel my hair appointment." I fake coughed into the phone for emphasis. "I've unexpectedly come down with the flu."

"No, I'd better not reschedule at this time, thanks. I'll have to call back."

"No, I'm sorry, Taren. This weekend's not going to work for us. We have other plans."

"No, it's okay, Ash, thanks for offering. I'll go on my own. You know how I get carsick."

"Hey, I'm sorry to cancel last minute, Kina. I woke up not feeling well. I think I'm sick."

"Maybe see you next weekend?"

"I'll stop by another time."

But then, I never did.

I'd become agoraphobic.

I cried and trembled, my stomach churning at the thought of having to do things most people wouldn't think twice about. I refused to get into a car with a friend—the thought of not being in control, not being able to get away or find a bathroom, terrified me. I avoided any place with a rigid time requirement, like movie theaters or hair and nail salons. My hair grew halfway down my back because I was too afraid to leave the house to get it cut.

I would only go out if absolutely necessary, and provided it fell within my parameters. I had to be in my own vehicle, and I had to take both Imodium and Dramamine in advance. In fact, I always carried an assortment of medications with me, and I double-checked and triple-checked I had Ativan in my purse at all times. I hovered my hand over it reassuringly, guarding it; its sequestered presence always a small comfort.

But for the most part, I just hid in the ugly yellow house, afraid to leave what had become my safe space for fear of having a panic attack—or, worse yet, shitting my pants—an intrusive thought I couldn't get out of my head.

The Paxil I had been taking on and off since university clearly wasn't working, so I drugged myself up with Imodium and Dramamine to get to the nearest clinic. One of the doctors there prescribed me Lexapro instead, claiming it would be more effective, but all that changed in the coming weeks was my weight. And as someone who'd never had to worry about their weight before, I didn't know what to do.

People told me it was basic math, calories in and calories out, so I started tracking everything. I bought a food scale and weighed my portions, decreasing my meal sizes a bit further every week. Yet running on the treadmill continued to get harder, as each week, my knees told me I was still gaining more weight.

After three months of taking Lexapro, gaining thirty pounds, and not feeling any better, I decided I was done with it. I refused to take another dose. I didn't call the prescribing doctor or my new shrink. I didn't read the instructions on the bottle on how to appropriately wean myself off. Instead, I quit cold turkey.

Vertigo, dizziness, and brain zaps that made me feel like I was short-circuiting soon followed. And even though the internet told me that these side effects would clear up in two to six days, they continued for several months.

I could no longer run; I couldn't even walk Pete. I was so disoriented that I had to hold onto walls so that I wouldn't fall over. And to make matters worse, those pills opened up a part of my brain that had never been opened before—they'd created synapses that couldn't be undone.

I knew exactly how the Diagnostic and Statistical Manual of Mental Disorders described a major depressive episode—I'd read countless case studies while pursuing my bachelor's degree in psychology. But that's all they ever were to me, stories and statistics. I'd personally never experienced anything like it; that is, until the day the lights simply turned off.

I lay on our black leather couch as days turned into weeks, and weeks turned into months, with zero recollection of what I did or even thought during that time.

I wasn't sad, I didn't cry—I was exhausted, in a way I'd never experienced before. It was as if I was absent from my body, absent from my mind even. Like the essence of who I was ceased to exist. I didn't think, I barely spoke. I hardly even noticed Marty leaving for work in the mornings or coming home at the end of each day.

Inside of me, there was a great nothingness. I was empty. Apathetic and nearly catatonic. Yet two out of my only five friends in Pittsburgh got mad at me during that time (one doing it slightly more politely than the other).

"What's going on? Where have you been?" Taren demanded, fight and fury ringing clear in her voice the second I picked up the phone.

"Um, I don't know. I guess I've been here," I said, not really sure how much time had passed since I'd last seen my friends. I wasn't even sure of the current day or month.

"Well, you haven't called. I haven't seen you. Are we okay? Are we even *friends* anymore?"

"Yeah, of course we are," I said quickly, not understanding why girls always had to jump to that.

I'd watched them ask those types of questions my entire life, and it had always felt unnecessarily dramatic. How they made it about them and their insecurities—treating friendship like it was something so fragile it was sure to break at any moment. I wondered why it never occurred to them that the issue may be outside of them, outside of the friendship even, and that there might be something bigger going on.

"I guess I haven't been feeling well," I admitted, tears starting to well up in my eyes. I felt a sudden flash of hope, thinking that maybe someone *had* noticed what was happening to me, but she immediately cut back in.

"I've been going through stuff, too."

I recoiled from the phone, shocked at her vitriol. "Uh, I'm sorry," I said, fumbling for words as a rush of emotions washed over me, guilt predominantly. Maybe this wasn't about insecurities, not going shopping or out for lunch. Maybe I'd let her down somehow. Maybe she, too, could be dealing with something big.

"Well, you've been a bad friend," she snapped. And then she hung up the phone.

I stared at the dead receiver in my hands, then I slowly placed it back on its charger. I was unaware of what I was even doing as I made my way upstairs to my bedroom on instinct. I entered my closet, shut the door behind me, and dropped to the floor where I proceeded to sit in the darkness and cry. Hiding among the mess of our hanging clothes, I was wracked by big, ugly sobs.

When I was finally empty, I gathered myself up and called my best friend Christie. She had always seen me—we were one and the same, she and I—our connection immediate and easy. I felt a little better after having told her what had happened. But when weeks passed and nothing changed with my health, Taren and Kina both extricated themselves from my life. Neither one of them ever spoke to me again.

Pete stayed with me. We dozed on the couch together with HGTV on in the background, neither of us watching. It was nice that I had him and I didn't have to be alone. He and Marty were the only ones who truly understood.

We had to sleep during the day because at night, I was plagued by insomnia, restless legs, and drenching night sweats. I constantly woke cold and wet to find I'd soaked through both my pajamas and the sheets. I'd get out of bed, change my clothing and the bedding, only to wake a few hours later, finding it had happened yet again.

I didn't tell anyone about it, assuming it had to be my hormones. Instead, I drugged myself once again with Dramamine and Imodium to get back to the clinic for a different contraceptive prescription, neglecting to mention the embarrassing reason why.

Then my neck became stiff and started cracking, and my face erupted with swollen red pustules layered on top of more pustules. It hurt to smile or talk, and the pustules would sometimes crack and bleed when I did. So I drugged myself once again with Dramamine and Imodium and forced myself out of the house to see a dermatologist, going back and forth for stronger and stronger steroid creams, but it only kept getting worse.

I remember trying not to think about it as I lay on the couch during the day. And again as I ate my dinner in silence. I really tried not to think about it as I ran myself a bath, hoping the warm water would soothe both my inflamed skin and my desperately sad soul. I wasn't thinking about it at all as I stepped into the warm water and sank as best I could into the strange triangular corner tub, the yellow walls I hated so much all around me.

I wasn't thinking about the painful rash on my face. My cracking neck. My stomach. The insomnia, restless legs, and drenching night sweats. The loss of my friends. The depression or the anxiety. The vertigo, dizziness, brain zaps. I wasn't thinking about any of that at all when I saw it—my reflection in the chrome of the tub overflow plate.

I was fat. There were rolls, and my face was bleeding again, and I cried.

I couldn't help it.

I sat up, brought my knees up to my chest, and wrapped my arms around them, hugging them into me as I hung my head. And I sat there, all alone in the water, and I cried some more.

My issues all seemed completely unrelated to one another, out of my control, and inexorable. I was broken when, only months prior, I'd been whole.

I couldn't understand why.

EMPTINESS

I am so tired, yet I can't sleep.

Everything is throbbing.
My entire body is throbbing.

I'm so tired, I could cry.

I want to cry.
But I'm so tired, I don't even have the energy to cry.

I rarely write anymore. Time has passed, but I can only remember snippets. Barely conscious, I'm enduring a level of sick I hadn't previously known was even possible.

I spend every day here in bed—my body inert, unable to get up, unable to even roll over. The pain has completely overtaken me, incapacitated me. I am being stabbed, pinched, and crushed in every part. The pain drains me, the medication drains me, this illness has taken all that there was of me.

Now, there is nothing left.

I stare at the blank wall beside me for most of the day, too debilitated to do anything else, like read or watch TV. Weeks' worth of unread text messages pile up on my phone that I don't even attempt to check, let alone respond to. So dead tired, so utterly and completely destroyed, I can't even think.

I am uncomfortably short of breath, breathing so shallowly that there is little to no movement left in me at all; it seems my body is so worn out that it barely even bothers to breathe.

I don't eat. I don't even remember the last time I drank water.

The days pass, yet nothing changes.

I do not move. I cannot move. My body refuses to move.

Hours go by, and I do not sit up. I do not roll over. I'm vaguely aware of my pain, though I don't bother to try and move to avoid it. I occasionally wonder if my body might be deteriorating even further from this lack of movement, but my mind is so foggy with fatigue, I can't think clearly enough to tell.

It doesn't matter.

I'm so consumed by lassitude, nothing matters.

This is how I am now. Every day, unmoving, barely alive. The days fade together, and I have little to no memory of any of it. My mind goes in and out of a trance-like state, a semi-conscious coma. Awake or asleep, no one is quite sure. Not even me.

Marty checks in on me, but I am unresponsive. I hear him come in. I hear him as if I'm frozen in sleep. My eyes are even open as I stare at the white wall beside me—yet I don't see it, just as I don't see him.

I don't blink. I don't move. I don't respond. I lie like this every day.

My body and my mind alike are shut down. Thoroughly depleted.

Even with all that I should be worried about, all that I still need to solve, my mind remains blank.

I am a void.

TEXAS

TWENTY-NINE YEARS OLD

I healed myself in Texas.

At least, that's what I told everyone.

We moved to North Houston in the spring of 2012, after only eighteen months in Pittsburgh. As always, our belongings were transported in a twenty-six-foot-long moving truck as we headed out in our own vehicle—Marty at the wheel and Pete on my lap.

I was excited. Nervous but excited as we drove the fourteen hundred miles to our new state. I'd always loved the tropical parts of Texas and was in need of a change. And our expat friends would soon be transferred too, so we'd get to share the adventure with them.

The company had again rented us a house, this time an amazing five-thousand-square-foot Mediterranean that we'd picked out online. For two full days in the car, all we could talk about was our excitement. But when we arrived in person, eager to see the house for the very first time, we were devastated to discover its condition.

The house was only a few years old, yet every part was in disrepair. The paint was peeling, the appliances didn't work, everything was either loose or broken, and it was filthy—beyond anything we could have ever imagined. The walls were splattered with unidentifiable stains and sticky multicolored drips. The fridge had mold. Spider webs and mud dauber nests were in every corner. There was even a pile of dog shit on the carpet upstairs.

It wasn't a great welcome to our new state, and it definitely didn't feel like that house could ever be our home.

Professionals were brought in, and tense words were exchanged with both the realtors and the landlords. Everything had to be washed down and the carpets replaced; it took about a week to get it clean enough before I was even willing to move our stuff indoors.

It was a cool house though, and in a great location—the reason we had taken the gamble on renting it sight unseen. I immediately started to plug away at restoring it. Even if it was just a rental, I wanted it to feel like a home.

It was lakefront, in a gated subdivision on Lake Conroe, where everyone had their own private dock and pool. And as two kids originally from Saskatchewan, we were enamored with the idea that we'd be able to enjoy those things year-round.

We found Texas exotic. There was obviously no part of it that reminded us of back home in Canada, yet we loved it all the same. The gorgeous tropical landscape: palm trees, ginger, bougainvillea, and hibiscus. The shorebirds: blue herons, great white egrets, and roseate spoonbills. Through the windows, I loved watching the green anoles and tree frogs that climbed all over the glass, their suction-cupped fingers and transparent torsos displaying their tiny beating hearts. I even got a kick out of the elusive alligators and adjusted to the daily presence of wolf spiders and poisonous snakes—often finding them in our yard and even our garage. Texas, to me, was a tropical adventure. An entirely new world to explore.

I liked driving out to the Gulf with Pete and watching him run in and out of the surf, biting at the saltwater waves. I loved the serenity of living at that lake—watching the birds and swimming in the pool—it really was paradise. I even loved the warmth and coziness of the thick and humid tropical heat (despite having to be careful with my tendency to faint).

Healthwise, I was able to enjoy most of it. I had no explanation for the drastic change that had occurred in my health since leaving Pittsburgh, I only knew that I felt a lot better. Maybe not perfect yet, but I was back to getting out of the house every day and working. And I smiled a lot, even if I was still hiding some angst.

I felt motivated that my time in Texas—however brief it might be—should be my own. I knew what had happened to me in Pittsburgh wasn't exactly normal, and I didn't want to be held back by my health like that ever again. So, taking advantage of the little bit of health that I did have, I set out to find myself a new dermatologist almost right away, as well as a general practitioner.

After a few failed attempts with purely allopathic doctors, I ended up finding a woman online who was both trained as a medical doctor *and* a naturopathic one. It took me a full day to get up the nerve to call her, but when I did, I asked the receptionist over the phone if Dr. Song treated anxiety.

"Pardon me?" she asked.

I internally cursed my timidness. "Anxiety," I repeated a bit louder, cringing at the volume of my own voice. And then I left it at that, neglecting to mention any other symptoms. It was anxiety, after all, that was at the forefront of my mind.

On the day of the appointment, I took a handful of Dramamine and Imodium, packed my Ativan, and set off into the middle of nowhere to find the tiny old house-turned-medical office. I spent the entire drive deep breathing, bouncing in my seat with nerves, trembling, and crying a bit. But once inside the little foyer, I was met with love, and I sensed it right away. Both Annie, the receptionist I'd talked to on the phone, and Dr. Song were filled with genuine compassion.

"Welcome, welcome," Dr. Song greeted me in her thick southern accent as she gestured for me to follow her from the single chair in the waiting room across the hall to a private office. The entire building, it seemed, comprised no more than those two rooms. "I see you've got your paperwork all filled out, so we're all set on that," Dr. Song continued. "Now, before we get started, would you be comfortable with Annie and me praying with you?"

Her warmth was a bit unexpected, but her offer of prayer was completely so. It was out of my comfort zone, not having been raised in a particularly religious family, but I had gone to Catholic school so I knew how it worked. And I didn't want to be rude. I was there for help, after all—a little prayer couldn't hurt.

At my shy nod of acquiescence, Dr. Song called Annie into the little office, and the three of us huddled together—hands held, heads bowed. It was both extremely uncomfortable and equally beautiful at the same time. No one had ever prayed over me before, and here were these two strangers doing exactly that. Then Annie gave my hand a quick squeeze as she left the room, and I was left alone with Dr. Song to go through my intake forms.

It was time to admit my anxiety.

"We've moved around a lot," I said, staring down at my hands as I fidgeted, rubbing them together. "It's probably something simple. I mean, my life's been repeatedly uprooted, and so, I guess, I've felt unsettled as a result..." I wasn't sure what I was expecting from her, a prescription maybe; I'd only ever been to Western doctors. I certainly didn't expect her to care. Or give me more than ten minutes.

"I don't think so," Dr. Song said bluntly.

I looked up at her in surprise.

"I'd like for us to keep talking about that."

And so we did. We spent over an hour together that day as she dug deeper into my past. She wanted to know everything. Like where I lived and with whom. What I ate, when I ate, how I ate, and so on. And somewhere along the way, I became comfortable with her, finally admitting something that I'd kept private for much too long.

I'd had diarrhea nearly every day for close to *ten years* without ever telling anyone. Not even a doctor.

I was quick to explain that it hadn't started out that severe, but had gradually worsened—until, eventually, having diarrhea constantly, all throughout the day, every single day, had become my new normal. It was the reason I was there in her office—blaming it on anxiety, I assumed *that* was what was out of control and needed to be addressed.

Dr. Song, however, had a different theory.

She went on to teach me about the gut-brain connection and questioned whether the anxiety had given me diarrhea or if the constant daily diarrhea had given me anxiety. An important distinction and something I hadn't ever considered.

With her help, I started tracking my symptoms in relation to my diet. And through testing in the subsequent weeks and months, we discovered that in addition to some food sensitivities, I did have leaky gut and celiac disease. I started a GAPS diet right away—eliminating gluten, dairy, sugar, eggs, alcohol, coffee, processed foods, and more than thirty other items.

No longer on Lexapro, the weight started to fall off of me. I healed my gut and the unexplained rashes, and the agoraphobia and depression soon became a distant memory.

I threw out the food scale and ate as much as I wanted.

I lost over fifty pounds.

Feeling fantastic, I started running again. I loved hitting the open road with my strong body carrying me forward—the pulse of my music coming through my earbuds, the metronome for my legs. It was the first time I'd been able to run comfortably, completely pain-free, since my knee surgery in my teens.

I cut my hair into a pixie—I'd lost some of it on my healing journey, and this was a style I'd long admired but been too scared to pursue, just not for the reasons anyone would think. I knew a cut like that required regular maintenance, and I'd been too anxious to frequent the salon. Committing to an appointment every five weeks was a huge milestone for me, an indication that I was healed.

I didn't shed a single tear as my long, natural hair was all cut off. Rather, I felt liberated to rid myself of my previous life and the angst that had held me back from so much. I donated all twenty-six inches of hair that day in memory of our sweet Kristin, who'd found wigs so helpful when fighting cancer at such a young age.

I looked and felt like a new person, confident with my weight loss and a platinum-blonde pixie—but not everyone responded positively to my transformation.

"Is that a wig?" one friend asked.

"You better not lose any more weight," threatened a family member.

"You looked better before," another felt the need to tell me.

And a lot of distrust: "Stomach issues? Sure." Followed by exaggerated eye rolls. "I guess that's why you're so skinny now. You never eat."

I knew it was my own fault that people didn't understand my weight loss; I'd hidden years of symptoms, both mental and physical. Up until then, I'd only ever told the world that I was okay—better than okay. I'd only ever shown the world that my life was perfect. But even if it was my own fault that my friends and family hadn't known my entire medical history, I still found it embarrassing that they didn't believe me now.

I felt judged, and I shut down a bit—not liking the attention. Self-conscious about having to defend myself, and having a few too many awkward conversations about chronic diarrhea, I no longer wished to disclose anything about my health.

I knew I wasn't anorexic, and that was all that mattered. But my body had become so sensitive to food that I had become afraid of eating the "wrong" foods or "bad" foods. In my desperation and dedication to be cured of my ailments, I'd inadvertently stumbled into orthorexia. I'd become extreme, obsessed with perfect nutrition, yet after all the recent judgments, I didn't think I could talk to anyone about it.

I knew I was too thin—my bones were hurting, and I was finding it difficult to sit in chairs or sleep at night. Yet I truly believed that the healthier lifestyle was working wonders for me. It seemed that being too thin was better than constant daily diarrhea. Too thin was better than too heavy and unable to run. And too thin was certainly better than agoraphobia and depression.

I was absolutely willing to put up with a few side effects of "too thin" for all the progress I had made.

I didn't worry that sometimes carrying a purse caused such intense pain and spasms for me that it would take days for me to recover. I didn't worry that I had near-fainting spells on a daily basis. Or that I didn't outgrow my motion sickness; rather, it only continued to grow in severity. Or even that my body, head to toe, would regularly break out in a rash. And so I didn't worry when I suffered an injury out on one of my runs either—a sudden and sharp pain in my tailbone that caused my right thigh to go numb.

I assumed the latter was my sciatic, and I didn't tell anyone about it. It was important to me that my story be clear moving forward: My problems were a thing of the past. I was now healed. I was okay.

I did feel healed, even the first time I peed my pants. It shocked me, but I assumed the loss of control must have been the result of a mild bladder infection, because I felt great otherwise. I didn't bother telling anyone about it or even go see a doctor; I assumed it would go away on its own.

But it didn't.

I wasn't consistent. I could hold my urine for hours when, out of nowhere, I would get an uncontrollable urge and not be able to make it to the bathroom in time. It was totally embarrassing. I'd previously heard older women complain about bladder issues and started to assume it was a sign of my aging. But at twenty-nine years old, I was pretty sure I was the only one of my friends with any of these problems.

I was ashamed that I couldn't get my life under control. I didn't know anyone more dedicated to their health and nutrition, and yet I knew I still wasn't entirely well. In many ways, I felt inferior for it. Inadequate. I was unable to bring myself to admit that I'd been trying so hard and still wasn't succeeding.

Desperate to move on and desperate to be normal, I pushed this symptom to the back of my mind, along with all of the others. I made a conscious decision to see my issues as a speed bump; my health may have slowed me down temporarily, but it wasn't going to stop me. I had an athlete's mindset: always pushing through. I considered myself cured, and I credited Dr. Song—deciding that speed bump was forever in my rearview mirror.

I *needed* it to be in my rearview mirror.

Just as my health felt like a speed bump in my life, all of those relocations felt like a speed bump for my career. I was growing antsy—suddenly hyperaware of where I stood in comparison to those around me.

It's not that I regretted prioritizing Marty's career over mine when we'd moved to the States; it had obviously been the right choice for us financially and a decision we'd happily made together. I was proud of the life we'd built—grateful for the chain of events and experiences we never would have been blessed with had we stayed at our previous jobs in Canada. But while I had assumed there would be challenges, I hadn't fully understood the implications of our decision. Or the sacrifice I was making.

I had been young, and as it turned out, those years were integral to actualizing my self-confidence. I felt it in my career, though also on some level as I was becoming an adult—I felt left behind.

Marty and our expat friends all worked in the corporate world, and with each passing year, I'd watched the rift between our lives grow. Their corporate world sparkled with wealth—all-expense paid business trips, extravagant dinners, and tickets to shows—and my career had never offered any of that. They wore fancy clothes and designer shoes and commuted in luxury sports cars to shiny, all-glass office buildings. By contrast, I worked independently from home, often wearing sweatpants and covered in drywall dust on the days I spent out on site.

They'd long since established themselves and become successful, already holding impressive titles like senior manager and director, when I was perpetually just getting started. I had a work history that felt embarrassingly broken up. And as they all spoke the same corporate language, discussing their coworkers and bosses, bonuses, investments, and 401Ks, I sat silently with nothing of my own to contribute. I was an outsider, an observer of their very grown-up conversations. It wasn't hard to see that everyone had long surpassed me and my self-printed business cards with the simple title of designer.

The ironic part was that these same people often hired me, needing me to draw blueprints and design their fancy homes, yet I still saw them as so much further ahead than me. It was obvious they were on the fast track to achieving Western society's ultimate definition of success—power, prestige, and wealth—when I was just their hired help.

It made me question myself, my role in my marriage, and my value. And the outdated sexist culture surrounding me in Texas only fed into those doubts.

I'd followed my man. This was my fourth major move; we were in our seventh house in only nine years of marriage. All along, I had chosen to prioritize and follow his career, allowing mine to be secondary. Allowing myself to be secondary. And I worried that, on some level, maybe I'd taken the easy way out. Maybe I should have been striving for more all that time.

I didn't want to be a guest in his sparkly world. Though it had never even occurred to me to desire wealth or status before, I knew now that I didn't want to be seen simply as someone's pretty wife. I wanted to be smart, successful, and impressive on my own accord. But as I found myself standing in the background behind his career, in the shadows of his success, and on the fringe of the glamor of the corporate world that intimidated me so much, I found I didn't measure up.

I questioned whether design had been the right career choice, unsure if I would ever be able to find comparative success. I fought against the societal stigma surrounding working from home and not having a "real" job. And as I saw that many unaccredited women liked to call themselves interior designers just because they liked decorating, I constantly defended against that assumption, too.

I wondered if I should have been an architect or an engineer instead, as I'd excelled easily in all those advanced classes in school. I regretted which interior design program I'd taken, never admitting that after my bachelor's degree, all I had were a few diplomas. I never said it outright, but I definitely alluded to the fact that I held a more prestigious second degree.

I was a fraud—and I had no excuse for it. I was the least successful out of all of my friends and family, and I didn't even have any children. Then, one by one, as I watched all of my friends become moms, I felt left behind there, too.

I wasn't sure where I fit in anymore, and I questioned what value I even brought to the table. I was spiraling, slowly losing track of my purpose and identity. I felt that if I wasn't equally successful, if I wasn't needed in some way, whether career-wise or as a mother, then I didn't even know who I was, let alone what I was worth.

I'd succeeded in everything I'd ever pursued in life. I'd always won. And though I never would have had the audacity to word it as such, I'd always inwardly identified as a winner.

I wasn't winning anymore.

In my mind, I blamed our relocations, the choice to put my career second, and the glamor of the corporate world. But it wasn't nearly as simple as that.

I was hiding the fact that I still felt amiss. Not just physically, but mentally, too. There was a fog that kept rolling in, a paranoia. Something underlying, thoughts I couldn't place, and emotions I couldn't control. Something I was always fighting to hide—something I was simply fighting.

I didn't have the words for it, but I felt a bit broken inside. Different. Maybe I'd never felt entirely normal—I'd always been told that I was "too sensitive," that I needed to "toughen up, girl," and so at some point in my youth, subconsciously, I had done just that. Yet after years of successfully hiding this mysterious, undesirable emotion away, I could feel it bubbling to the surface again. Was this just sensitivity? Insecurity? Or was this something else? Something *bigger*? I feared I was becoming unstable.

I tried again.

I built a shield of perfectionism around me to protect myself from my own "sensitivity." It was my attempt to outwork and outsmart ever feeling insecure or inadequate ever again. I wanted my health, my career, and my relationships to appear perfect—to be perfect—and I couldn't tolerate anything less. It was my way of taking control. My way of making sure people would like me. My way of making sure *I* would like me.

I wasn't purposely hiding my medical situation from my close friends and family; it was more that I was choosing to hide it from myself. I didn't want to be sick, so I lied to those around me. I lied to myself. I hid my symptoms, hid what my body was doing to me, and I forced myself to move on.

I was missing the crucial difference between having a positive attitude and living in denial.

I busied myself, chasing one distraction after another—accomplishing, always accomplishing—never allowing myself to sit with any of my fears. I portrayed an easy confidence, even though it was the furthest thing from the truth. Always saying things like "all good" and "no worries," I was desperate to appear laid-back—when deep down, not a single thing was all good, and I was nothing but worries.

An existential angst haunted me as I frantically pursued goal-based achievements, trying to find my purpose. Believing that my value could only be determined by what I accomplished and how well I accomplished it, I *needed* to get back to winning.

Marty was traveling internationally and working incredibly long hours, so I matched them. I didn't say a word about it, but I fabricated a system inside my head that somehow gave me a sense of equality despite our differing incomes. I not only worked as a successful interior designer, at times working more than seventy hours a week, but I insisted on becoming the best possible wife, too.

I ran the errands, got the groceries, and cooked every meal from scratch. I hosted our friends and family nearly every single weekend as if I were running a B&B. I was the only person in our entire gated community who had a full-time job, no maid, and mowed their own lawn in the hot Texas heat.

I had to do it all, and I had to do it myself. It was a compulsion; still, it didn't help. As time went on, and I saw the chasm only continue to grow between my work and the successfully glamorous careers of others around me, my insecurities grew along with it.

I doubled down again, swearing no one would be as busy as I was, as independent, as capable—I would succeed at that. And I refused to hire out any task that, with the help of the internet, I could learn to do myself. I learned to fix things, learned to build—I learned to do it all.

I volunteered at the Humane Society and built houses for Habitat for Humanity. I was also that friend, that neighbor who always offered to help, to babysit, to make a meal, or to spend several hours hanging someone's artwork on her day off. I took on more at work, too, breaking into the more lucrative side of the business with commercial design. I worked seven days a week and into every evening, all the while researching the master's degree program in architecture at Rice University and looking for homes to flip. It still wasn't enough; I felt I could have still been doing more.

We eventually bought some waterfront property on which I designed our very own lake house. I acted as the architect, not only drawing the blueprints, but managing the year-long construction. It was the most difficult yet most rewarding thing I'd ever done. A dream project for me, and the result a dream come true.

The house was a contemporary take on the popular Mediterranean, with a 1920s-inspired elegance. It was an enormous two-story with a soft gray stucco exterior, a dark chocolate clay-tile roof, and a soaring square-arch entrance clad in ivory travertine. A manicured tropical landscape surrounded it, and custom copper gas lanterns continuously burned, flanking the entrance through a private gated courtyard.

It was grand, spacious, and airy, with excessively tall ceilings, large windows, and oversized hallways and doors. Nothing short of opulent. It featured unnecessarily lavish details like three thousand square feet of uninterrupted vein-cut marble floors, rich espresso-stained solid wood doors and trim, oversized crystal chandeliers, and crystal doorknobs on gleaming chrome backplates. It was the epitome of luxury.

The kitchen was pure white, showcasing custom cabinetry and designer commercial-grade appliances, while oversized lanterns hung above a massively sprawling island. It gleamed. The backsplash was Moroccan glass, and the countertops were an imported Brazilian white Macaubas—vein-cut to match the marble floors, and three times the standard thickness with a mitered waterfall edge. A prestigious Putnam rolling library ladder even ran along the perimeter of the room, providing access to the highest bank of cabinets, and the center of the twelve-foot tray ceiling was clad in an espresso-stained hardwood, adding a necessary richness and warmth to the space.

If that wasn't enough, the adjacent open-concept family room boasted a palatial twenty-four-foot tall ceiling—the tray inset with that same solid hardwood, and an extravagant sixty-inch orb chandelier hung in the very center. The fireplace was white quartzite, the furniture designer, and the art oversized. Although, the true pièce de résistance was the backdrop to this magnificent space—an entire wall of windows looking out to a tropical landscape and an infinity-edge pool that appeared to flow straight into the lake beyond.

It was a stunning sightline.

Yet beyond the infinity pool, it continued.

Our private dock ran the entire width of our property where, at any time, we could stand-up paddle, jet-ski, or lower our newest MasterCraft into the water and cruise away with the music pumping, Pete on my lap, and the wind in our hair.

It was more than a fancy house.

It was a lifestyle.

And like an all-inclusive resort, I made sure to keep it immaculate at all times. I kept the marble floors polished and the crystal gleaming, the yard pristine, the grass perfectly cut and edged, the tropical flowers always in bloom, and the pool the most precise shade of aqua.

I did it without any help. And I didn't stop there.

I kept the bar and kitchen fully stocked, and made food and drinks steadily—hand delivering it out to our guests poolside. I didn't mind it; in fact, in many ways, I liked taking care of our home and our guests. I took pride in it. I loved sharing a place that meant so much to us, as our dream home at the lake really was extraordinary. Even by Texas standards.

We had a life beyond anything I'd ever imagined, and there was maybe a part of me that needed that to be noticed. I couldn't help but be pleased to see in our guests' faces when it was. I saw it in their reactions upon arrival at the house, in the way their necks craned upward as they gawked around, and, especially, in the things that they said.

"Whoa."

"I've never been in a house like this before."

"How tall are those ceilings?"

"How big is that chandelier?"

"Ben tripped right into me, he was so captivated looking around."

"I hope you don't mind that Tim took some pictures to show his family while you were outside. He even FaceTimed his sister!"

Marty and I talked about it, too, often reminiscing about how much our lives had changed since moving to the States. We talked about how much we had grown as individuals, as well as a couple. The places we'd been and the things we had seen. And how far we'd come financially, from the people we'd been not so long ago—distraught over the unforeseen cost of repair when a cherry pit had gotten lodged inside the dishwasher.

Now we were only half joking when we called our home a château. I carried designer handbags and Marty wore designer shoes, and we drove Porsches and had perfect tans year-round. Thin, blonde, and beautiful—the perfect couple—Ken and Barbie people had even called us.

Our life really was exceptional, and our home absolute perfection. I knew it, because I'd curated every last detail of them both. And as we sat with our guests in the luxuriously elegant great room—surrounded by all of that marble and crystal, and looking out onto our very own tropical paradise—our obvious success couldn't be ignored. Yet as I looked around at our guests' faces, their expressions of awe and obvious impress, it seemed I'd managed to convince everyone around me, except myself.

Despite everything, I didn't feel like a success at all.

DEATH

"I'm going to die."

"You're *not* going to die."

It's a conversation we just keep having—me on text and Marty aloud. I'm saying it, but I'm not really saying it. I'm tiptoeing around it, being vague, not saying what I actually mean. Afraid to hurt him, I always let the conversation end there.

The reality is that the severity of my symptoms has had me facing my own mortality for quite some time now. And it's hard to explain what that feels like—when an illness has taken over every part of you. How you instinctively know that your body is no longer your own, and neither is your mind. Every part of you is so riddled with disease that you are more of it now than of your real self.

Recently a shift has occurred, and that's proving even harder for me to explain. I can feel it—the energy has seeped from my cells, my mind is slow, my body no longer moves, and my organs are failing. My body has shifted into a survival mode; the only functions left in me are reptilian. I breathe, and my heart beats, but at the rate I'm going, I have little confidence that I'll even be able to count on those much longer.

This isn't working.

It's been nineteen months since my life, as I'd once known it, ended in Hawaii. And despite my best efforts and commitment to a nearly year-long treatment, I haven't made any progress. This can't be Lyme—this isn't Lyme—because the treatment for it isn't working. I know it. I feel it. So when I say, "I'm going to die," or "My life will not be continuing on like this," I am saying those things with certainty.

If something doesn't happen soon, I'm going to kill myself.

That is what I'm trying to say.

And I don't say it to get attention, nor is it my intent to sound dramatic. In fact, by the time anyone reads this, it will all be over. I'm done trying to get help; I tried that for years, tried a few different antidepressants and several different therapists. Committed to a mental health routine: proper exercise, nutrition, and sleep. I even used my few daily allotted words to confide in a few of my trusted people, yet none reacted particularly concerned.

My friend gave me a blank, emotionless stare, and then she moved on as if I hadn't said anything alarming at all. The Lyme-guy told me he was supposed to commit me for a seventy-two-hour involuntary psychiatric hold but wasn't going to do that because I "sounded okay." And my psychologist Dr. Cathy did a lot of talking, but not a lot of listening—rushing to tell me that I wouldn't fit the qualifying criteria for an involuntary psych hold unless I had a suicidal plan. Yet oddly, Dr. Cathy did not ask me, not even once during our hour-long appointment, if I actually had a plan.

Since then, I've tried joining an online suicide support group, drafted a number of texts asking for help, and spent a long while staring at the number for the hotline—my finger hovering over the call button. But just as I never sent those texts, I never could bring myself to make the call. Because it turns out I don't want help for my depression anymore—I want to be cured of this disease. And if I can't? Then I do want to die.

Of course, I have a plan.

I've considered tying a noose and hanging myself from the pull-up bar mounted in our basement. On the few occasions I've been outside making my way into appointments, I've contemplated throwing myself into oncoming traffic—and with each car that passed, I dreamed how quickly it could all be over if I just pretended to trip.

A surgically sharp X-ACTO knife could also probably do it. I would have to slice upward on the vein in my wrist, or better yet, the carotid artery in my neck—though admittedly, I've been too repulsed by the thought of that gore.

I've spent most of my time staring at pill bottles, trying to calculate how many it would take to make it all end. But the inexactitude of that method always makes me a bit nervous, and for this, I need a guarantee. So I ended up researching *that*, and I settled on pills for euthanasia.

My plan is also to see my family once more. Though, obviously, I'm too unwell to travel up to Canada at this exact moment, and the borders are still closed, ultimately, I recognize that I'm far from being at my best. I'm scared to see my family like this, terrified I'd end up ruining the whole perfectly planned thing. I need to have control over my last visits, my last words, and those final hugs. I need those final memories to be perfect and complete for all of us.

Now is not the time for the perfect ending that I want.

In the meantime, I've been teaching Marty to cook. Confined to my bed, I lie here in the semidarkness with my laptop and used tissues as I dig deep into what little cognition I have left, writing out step-by-step instructions for the basics. I want him to still eat well after I'm gone.

I've also been composing my Last Will and Testament, hoping some guidance will help those I leave behind (like what I'd like them to do with my personal effects, my jewelry, art, and handbags). I don't believe in wasting money or ground space on fancy burials, and I'm not one for large gatherings or being the center of attention. I'd actually prefer not to have a formal funeral at all. Something simple might be nice; the smaller, the better, like my ashes spread somewhere in nature. Most importantly, I just don't want people to gather around and pretend I was perfect when we all know I was not.

I'm writing personal farewells to address some of this, but so far, I'm struggling to find words capable of expressing the great depth of my sorrow, remorse, and despair. The drafts sit unfinished, my letters incomplete. My explanations, my apologies. The magnitude of my love remains unwritten.

It seems that words are just words, and though my tears flow steadily, nothing I write manages to capture the depth of what I am feeling. The chaos in my mind and the weight in my heart are so much bigger than any words. Just like when I tried to write a simple goodbye on Kristin's beautiful casket, words, which have always meant so much to me, are completely insufficient again.

What is a word anyway, but a string of letters? And no string of letters could ever convey the depth of this shame or the limitlessness of the love I have for my family.

These journals may be all that I end up leaving behind—and I hate that. My family deserves so much more than this. I can only hope that in reading them, they'll someday understand why it was so important that I protect them.

Instead of doing good with my life, I've done nothing but cause sadness and pain. So now I must go.

I'm doing this all for them—I do hope they'll be able to see that. Some say actions speak louder than words anyway, and I did try my best. I tried to be strong, and I fought so hard to beat this illness. I fought every day to stay alive, not for myself, but for them. All of my efforts, my Herxing, my pains have been for them. Wanting to be better for them. To be healthy, to be happy. Wanting to have a future *with them*. Even though I was not strong enough, my best not good enough, I did try with everything I had.

Now my suicide will be for them.

I should be allowed to choose this—without accusations of selfishness and mutterings of "such a shame"—my life should be my own choice. I don't see any point in continuing to drain our finances on a mysterious illness with no cure and no medical support. I am, at this point, only a burden and an obligation, and it would be unfair of me to continue to subject my family to this misery. My sad existence here only hurts them. And while I hate to think of the heartache I will leave behind, I am devastated by the heartache I'm currently causing—that's ultimately what helped me decide.

I will not continue to expose anyone to this suffering and anguish any longer. My family will be better off without me; I can see that now. I can see it all. With time, they will be able to move on, and they will laugh again without the heavy dark cloud of my illness and failures hanging overhead. The kindest thing I could ever do, the greatest act of love I could possibly give, will be my own death.

One final act to free myself from this pain would also save them—from me.

I'm going to die.

It's not what anyone imagines for their life. And obviously, I don't want this disease, or suicide, to be what people remember about me. I hate that I'll be another statistic: among the 43.5 percent of people thought to have Lyme disease that are suicidal, and one of the 1,200 each year who actually commits the act.

I hate that it is ending like this.

I had so much more left to do.

I wanted to travel and see more of the world. Have a more successful career. Design more. Create more. There are blueprints in my head that have only made it half of the way onto paper, designs for custom furniture, and a house we haven't yet had a chance to build. I wanted to volunteer more. Help more. Connect more. I wanted to have children—the longing and the ache of *that* still haunts me. And with the borders remaining closed, I don't know if I'll get a chance to see my parents and JJ again.

I can't even think about leaving them and my Marty.

I wanted to love them more.

There are so many things I haven't done, haven't yet said. Things I've done wrong that I meant to make right. But I know it's already too late.

I don't recognize myself in the girl who writhes on the floor in pain. Who hides in the dark, tormented by anxiety, alone and heartbreakingly lonely, terrified of her own outbursts—yet explodes anyway, despite the precautions she had taken. Completely losing herself in the act, so filled with self-hate that she lashes out at her loved ones. Cruelly pushing them away during the times when she needed them the most.

I've lost myself.

I handle the fear. I am even learning to handle the pain. The anxiety. The depression. But I cannot handle that this disease, that I, have hurt my loved ones.

I am *not* who I once was.

I am no longer me.

That is the worst part of all.

So when Marty tries to console me—saying I'm "*not* going to die"—his words, intended to comfort, feel instead like a life sentence. A curse that I cannot escape. I am not yet *allowed* to go, even though my heart and my mind have already decided.

I want to die.

And I am ready.

In fact, I am no longer afraid of death. I am afraid of having to continue on like this, wishing for death every single day for the rest of my life. I am afraid of what I have become, but even more afraid of the trajectory that I'm on. I'm afraid that someday I might lose the last remaining true authentic pieces of me—my morals and values and the love and connection I have with my family. I'm afraid of the hurt I would inevitably inflict and the relationships I would most certainly destroy—until no part of me is recognizable, not even to myself.

I am not afraid of death.

I'm afraid of not getting out in time.

PETE

THIRTY-TWO YEARS OLD

Striving for more, I decided to join my business with an interior design firm in downtown Houston. There was one in particular I had in mind; it would be an hour's commute from the lake at least, but I'd been by their place many times, and thought it might be worth it.

    I printed my portfolio and walked into their office fairly spontaneously one day, requesting a meeting with the owner, Charlene. My goal was to work in a big office with other fun creatives, though I also saw the partnership as a way to acquire more clients. And Charlene would get the benefit of having an interior designer who could not only handle entire home designs but manage the office day to day.

    It sounded like a win-win.

    I was attracted to Charlene's energy when I first met her. She was a presence—a big woman with an even bigger personality, a dynamic charisma. She was magnetic. The type of person anyone would want to work with: warm, complimentary, and hilariously funny. I walked out after that first meeting excited about what our partnership would bring.

    Within the first week of working together, however, I learned it was all an act and the partnership a big mistake. As a transplant in Texas, I hadn't previously known that Charlene had such a terrible reputation around town. I was suddenly uncomfortable, unsure with whom I'd gotten myself, my business, and my reputation involved.

As warm and fun as Charlene could be, I saw she could be equally mean—two-faced the only way she knew. Complimenting an employee or a personal friend, or even one of her own children, she would then roll her eyes behind their backs and criticize them to me for hours in our shared private office.

She could be vicious, the head "mean girl."

Charlene made somebody cry every day at work. She blew up on a regular basis, screamed and swore abusively at the staff, and later sobbed and begged for their forgiveness—offering lavish gifts in an attempt to buy back their love and loyalty. She always claimed she was working on herself, but it never lasted.

She hired and fired people at a rate so extreme that I started keeping a list for legal reasons, should it ever come to that. Charlene thrived on drama, deliberately looking for something (or someone) to be outraged at each day and finding offense in absolutely everything.

She had big, bright, fiery red hair, and she wore flowy bohemian-style clothing, massively oversized on her already considerable frame. Both wild hair and dresses billowed behind her as she ran about the office—flapping her arms and squawking "911" over and over. She was a chicken with its head cut off, feathers floating down all around her.

Charlene was fifty-two years old and the star of her own dramatic world, full of daily tears and theatrics that even a teenage girl would be ashamed of.

I found her exhausting.

Yet, as stunned and horrified as I was to witness her behavior and complete lack of professionalism, I stayed—pushing aside my own intuition. I hoped that maybe I'd just caught her at an off time, and things wouldn't be as bad as they'd initially appeared. Not one to go back on my word, I wanted to give her the benefit of the doubt and our partnership a chance.

It got complicated after that, when two things occurred nearly simultaneously.

The first was that I realized I liked the other staff and didn't want to leave them alone with her. Things weren't as bad as I'd seen that first week—unfortunately, they were worse. However, I noticed I could help mitigate some of the issues, and the addition of my presence helped keep Charlene somewhat calm.

I liked that.

The second thing was that this allowed me to actually enjoy working there. I ran myself ragged, working seven days a week (five in the office and two in clients' homes). And the more I worked, the less Charlene even bothered to come into the office at all.

I liked *that* even more.

I loved being in charge. I was the one everyone always came to who could solve any problem, and the designer every client wanted to work with. It gave me a high. I spent my days in Texas designing homes bigger than anything I'd ever dreamed of. Homes that rivaled what I'd only seen in movies or *MTV Cribs*.

I was thriving.

After my first year of working downtown at Charlene's, I'd made so much money that I bought myself a brand-new Mercedes. I was on fire—the blip in my self-confidence from years prior was nothing but a distant memory. Not only was I back to winning again, I finally felt like a success.

Seeing this, seeing the value I'd brought to her business, Charlene insisted on befriending me. She invited me out for drinks to talk strategy, just us two. She called on me for help during family "crises" and important life events. She even invited Marty and me to join her family for special gatherings like Christmas and Easter.

She treated me differently than everyone else; she made me feel special and like I belonged. Like not only was I the partner, I was the best friend she'd always been searching for.

I started to let my guard down. Charlene didn't like anyone—and yet, she liked me. It felt like an ultimate win. But as in every *Mean-Girls*-type story, at some point, the bully always turns on her friend.

I guess I should have seen it coming.

Charlene blew up on me one day, demeaning me publicly in the middle of a staff meeting. Forgetting our initial agreement to be partners, she treated me instead like one of her abused employees. I tried to interject, tried to defend myself politely and respectfully, but she didn't allow me to get a word in.

She berated me and screamed at me in front of the staff for an hour. She cried. And flapped. And feathers flew. All the while, I waited silently, my jaw clenched, humiliated yet refusing to partake in her histrionics. I'd witnessed her do this too many times before, and I knew I hadn't done enough to stop her in the past; I'd felt guilty by association at that time. But now, I was paying the price for my fear-based passivity.

Charlene not only destroyed our year-long partnership that day but any chance at a friendship, too. I'd never be able to forget what she had done; despite her apologies and dramatic claims that she was working on herself, I knew I'd never be able to trust her again.

A few weeks later, Marty and I agreed to join some of his old work friends and start a new company in Colorado. The timing was perfect. I wouldn't have to get into any of the personal reasons why my partnership with Charlene couldn't continue. I wouldn't even have to see her around town anymore once we'd moved. It would be a clean and simple break, and my non-confrontational self loved the timing of it.

Charlene cried when I told her. "I can't do this without you!" she wailed. "Should I close altogether?"

"I'm sorry," I said. "It's nothing personal, it's that we're moving..."

"I can't do it alone," she interjected. "I can't do this. Should I close? Should I? Should I just close? What am I supposed to do? What am I supposed to do?"

I stood there with her in the empty office long after all the other employees had gone and listened to her ramble on. She never once asked about our move or Marty's new opportunity. She never brought up the fact that I was leaving my beloved lake house, though I'm not sure she'd ever paid enough attention to know its significance to me, anyway. She didn't show any interest at all in the major life event that was happening to me. It was, as it had always been, all about her.

By the next day, in a typical immature Charlene fashion, she stopped speaking to me altogether; she outright ignored me whenever we were in the same room. It wasn't until many days later that she addres sed me at all.

"You don't have to be here, you know," she hurled at me as she stomped past. And then she went back to ignoring me.

I disregarded her petulance, tense as it was, knowing as a professional I would never walk out with my work incomplete. I just spent my final weeks glued to my desk, focused on finishing up projects, tying up loose ends, and handing off work to other designers.

I had a lot going on; it might have been my fifth major move, but that didn't make it much easier. We were uprooting and changing our entire lives yet again; I didn't have the capacity for Charlene's drama, too.

Even though Marty and I had made the decision together, I was still in a bit of shock. It seemed like one day, we'd been talking theoretically about Denver, and the next day, I was packing—unsure what had happened to the mere weeks in between.

I had mixed feelings about it all. There was excitement for a new adventure, as well as some sadness. Our five years in Texas had been the longest by far that we'd ever lived somewhere, even if it was in three different houses. And it felt strange to be selling the lake house that I had so lovingly designed and built; I'd put a lot of myself into that home, three years of my time, energy, creativity, sweat, and tears. I wanted to have a massive going away party. I wanted to say a proper goodbye—not only to our neighbors, coworkers, and friends, but to that house.

Yet there was still so much to get done.

There was packing and cleaning and yard work, but I also had to stain the dock, clean the windows, and power wash the concrete all before the house could be photographed for the real estate listing. I had to find us a home in Denver and interview movers. I had to sell the boat and the sports car, the jet-ski and paddle boards, and our excess of oversized furniture—all the things we wouldn't be needing in Colorado.

It was a lot, and I was alone to accomplish it. I didn't want to bother Marty, who was somehow simultaneously finishing his Executive MBA, starting a new company, still working full-time for the old company, and living out in West Texas for the month, helping to close out a court case for work. Normally unfazed, this was the most stressed I'd ever seen him.

On top of it all, there was a tropical storm brewing out in the Gulf.

Following the storm preparedness checklist according to the County recommendations, I made sure we had extra batteries and filled the bathtubs with water. I stocked up on fuel, food, and essentials—shocked to see that the stores were already in short supply, many of the shelves completely bare. I added our life jackets to the kit, ensuring Pete's little life jacket and ID tag were in there as well. And finally, I hauled out the extra mattress to create a bunker in our closet—the only interior room without any windows in which we could hide—though I was sure it would never come to that.

We were no strangers to tropical storms in Houston and knew roughly what to expect. We never worried too much about it, but I was someone who liked to be prepared. Living in Texas *had* taught me that; it had given me a healthy reverence for the unpredictability and power of nature. And in Houston, I wasn't alone in that.

We all left work early on Thursday (on my second to last day), since the downtown offices were shutting down in anticipation of the storm. The nervous energy was infectious; everyone just waiting for it to hit and wondering how bad it would be. Wondering *what* it would be. Even Marty drove home for it, though that first morning was surprisingly pleasant.

In many ways, it was a welcome interlude from the stress we'd both been under the past few weeks. Both home from work together for the first time in a while, we spent the morning happily chatting while we packed the kitchen dishes. We stood side by side at the island as we watched the rain fall gently out the windows. It was nice.

It was only as the rain continued to fall into the afternoon that we eventually decided to abandon our packing in favor of preparing our property. We tied things down and hauled patio furniture inside, and then we did the same for some of our neighbors.

Overall it was a productive day—rainy, but not at all a big deal. Yet I was starting to get a weird feeling. The unknown of the impending storm still loomed, and I could feel the unspoken truth hanging heavy in the air.

The rain wasn't stopping.

We ate dinner and watched the storm worsen even further into the evening. We sat at the kitchen island and, without much else to do, we turned on the news and refreshed our weather apps.

The storm continued to worsen. And worsen.

We watched the news, and we refreshed our apps.

It worsened even further.

And further.

We refreshed the apps, we refreshed the apps, we refreshed the apps—until it was official. Our no-big-deal-rainy-day had become a big deal.

Hurricane Harvey was headed directly for us.

Things escalated quickly after that—with the storm hitting us on the second day, just like in all of those disaster movies I'd once loved. The wind howled. The rain fell in angry sheets. The trees all leaned over, and the always-calm bay of the lake behind our house turned to whitecaps.

The tornadoes started that evening with emergency alerts blaring repeatedly on our phones, jolting our already frazzled nerves. SEEK IMMEDIATE SHELTER NOW. Neighbors, friends, and family all panicked and texted and called, only adding to the chaos on our phones. They warned us each time another twister was in the area—and we rushed to check out the window.

The sound on the roof was a roar, constant and deafening, but the visibility out the windows was nil. So it was back into the bunker of our closet, away from the glass and away from the storm. We hid with Pete during each of the fifty tornadoes that visited the Houston area that night.

Never ones to worry too much about the weather, we could feel that this storm was different.

We woke with a start, early on the third day, with calls and texts from neighbors who needed help. The risk of tornadoes was over, but flooding was the new concern. Harvey hadn't continued on its predicted path throughout the night, rather, it had stayed—sitting above us, spinning and dumping rain at unprecedented rates.

Twelve inches of rain had been quickly surpassed by twenty-four. Then thirty-six. And the lake had risen significantly as a result—cresting over the banks, submerging the docks, and flooding the yards and pools. Boats and boat houses had been crushed in the night. Unsecured boats and debris now floated everywhere.

We geared up the best we could before running outside to help. Through the still-pouring rain, we waded through the flood, pulling and pushing boats to somewhat secure locations. We dove under the murky water as necessary and reaffixed the boats randomly to trees and fence posts, whatever we could find still exposed. Each home, each family with a completely different setup. A completely different set of challenges.

We spent the entire day like that, answering one distress call after another, and running out into the storm to help. We took care to avoid the masses of floating fire ants and kept watch for displaced water moccasins, alligators, and submerged electrical. Our garage was completely overtaken with each round of drenched clothing and rubber boots that had somehow disintegrated into unusable pieces.

Then we got the call.

"We don't know what to do," our neighbor Sam said, with distress and tears in his voice. "The water—I mean, the lake—it's lapping against our patio door."

"We'll be right there," Marty said, as he and I were already running to the mudroom to throw on our sneakers.

"We'll be right back, Petey," I called over my shoulder as we rushed out the door. Yet as we splashed over to their house, we realized we had no idea how we could possibly help.

Harvey had been classified as a major Category 4 hurricane, and catastrophic damage was expected.

That night, we lay in bed with no intention of sleeping. We hadn't been able to do anything to help Sam and his wife, and we were sick to our stomachs with worry. The foundation of our home was built only a few inches above Sam's—we knew we would be next.

We left the blinds open and the outdoor floodlights on as we stared out, watching as the rain continued to fall and the waters continued to rise. I cried on and off, huddled up with both Marty and Pete, watching through our beautiful picture windows the destruction that slowly crept toward us.

By two o'clock in the morning, flooding at our house was imminent. We were out of options. We got out of bed and started to carry all our packed boxes and furniture up to the second floor, one item after another. Boxes. Chairs. Side tables. Area rugs. Anything we could lift, we carried up the stairs together, silent and somber in the night. Then we went back to our bedroom, where we continued to sit and wait.

The waiting maybe was the worst part of all.

Running around and helping people had given us a false sense of control. Now without that distraction—just sitting and waiting, watching the dirty, angry stormwater approach our dream home—it was devastating. It had been a three-day, slow-motion nightmare, and we had reached the climax.

Overwhelmed with anxiety and grief, the three of us huddled together in front of the windows once more, keeping sentinel and praying that the water wouldn't enter our room. The hours passed. We tossed and we turned. But each time we checked out the window, we saw the water was indeed an inch closer.

I opened my eyes at dawn, just as the sun peeked over the horizon, its beautiful rays the first I had seen in days. I blinked. And blinked again, squinting into the light.

The rain had ceased.

The waters had stopped rising.

"No way," I whispered. And then I whooped, my cheers intentionally waking Marty. "Get up! Get up!"

I ran out of the bedroom, down the hallway, and burst out the patio door. Tears welled in my eyes as I rushed out across the covered lanai, with Marty and Pete right behind me. The three of us splashed out from under the roofline and tilted our faces up to the sun in relief.

Gratitude overwhelmed me—but it was short-lived, quickly replaced by survivor's guilt.

Homes, boats, and docks were destroyed. The ground, still covered in disgusting brown flood water, was littered with unrecognizable debris. Pieces of people's lives drifted past. Helicopters circled overhead. And I watched as the convoy of oversized military vehicles of the National Guard rolled in, one after another, in shades of khaki—like a scene straight out of a movie.

I shuddered. Swallowing down any joy or celebration, I felt instead only raw vulnerability at our extremely close call.

This was real.

We set out right away, looking to see if there was anywhere we could help. We didn't have to go very far—the houses around us were all destroyed, impossible for us to choose which was the worst. We'd only made it a block from home when we saw a group had gathered in front of one—nothing official, just neighbors who had come together in a crisis. And that felt like a good place to start.

A large boat lay on its side, in the middle of the front lawn, even though the lake was at the rear. I tried not to gawk at it as we approached, but there was no trailer, and it was much too large to have floated up between the houses. It didn't make any sense.

We had to walk around it in order to introduce ourselves. Trying to be respectful, I intentionally didn't look at the boat, and I kept my eyes focused on the task in front of me. Marty and I were assigned work in the living room, and we attempted to clean and restore what once had been. However, not even five minutes in, our efforts felt futile.

I could see directly through the walls, straight out to the still-turbulent lake beyond—the Sheetrock and siding had both been completely shredded. There wasn't a single pane of glass left in the once lovely windows; I could only guess that we were all standing on it. The hardwood floors must have existed somewhere beneath us, too, buried deep below several inches of lake water, mud, and debris.

My heart ached as I finally allowed myself to take it all in. The destruction. The volunteers. The homeowner and her daughter who stood off to the side in the corner of the room, out of everyone's way. I could see they were going through albums of soggy photographs, cataloging the memories by taking pictures on an iPhone. One after the other. They smiled through their tears at the memories, photographed them, and let the limp, saturated images fall into a growing pile of trash.

"It's her ninetieth birthday," I heard from beside me.

"Pardon?" I asked, turning to see the man who'd joined to watch the scene playing out.

"The homeowner," he said. "Today is her birthday. She turned ninety."

My heart ached a little more. And then we continued doing what we could for her, even though it wasn't enough.

We removed debris and cut out the waterlogged drywall from her home. We hauled huge broken sections of decking into trash piles at the curb. We were filthy—covered in mud and mysterious bug bites, scraped up and bleeding. Yet with each load we hauled outside, we saw that the streets around us were filling with mountains of remains as volunteers at every home attempted to make order out of the chaos. And as the community came together like that, it was somehow both heartwarming and devastating all at the same time.

A few more days of volunteering passed like that, and eventually, the waters receded. Grocery stores and gas stations reopened, and official restoration efforts got underway. The devastation in Texas was far from resolved, but life needed to continue on.

Marty drove back to the court case in West Texas, and I went back for my final day at Charlene's.

There was no going away party for me at work; rather, an uncomfortable heaviness hung in the air. Everyone was on edge after the hurricane, and we all tiptoed around Charlene who was still, after everything, unable to hide her anger at me for leaving.

"You don't have to be here," she snapped at me. But I stayed, feeling like it was the right thing to do. The office had flooded that weekend, and I knew they needed as many hands as possible to get the desks and samples out of the water.

It was another hard day—emotionally, as well as physically.

In the end, all the staff offered me were awkward promises to stay in touch and tentative goodbyes as they cast furtive glances over at Charlene, hoping she wouldn't overhear them being cordial. Then I left, feeling empty and incomplete as I walked out of that office alone for the very first time. We'd all always locked up and walked out together, but not on that day. Not ever again. I'd put my whole heart into that place for nearly two years, and *that* was how it ended.

I drove home solemnly, utterly drained from the hurricane and the drama at work. I immediately saw that Pete wasn't acting right—still not eating after the stress of the storm, and maybe even a bit lethargic. His stomach looked distended, too. Sick perhaps, though it wasn't for any obvious reason I could put my finger on. A bit unsteady, the difference in his gait was nearly imperceptible. Yet something about his movements seemed off. And it scared me.

With Marty back in court, I was left to ponder this alone. I knew Pete's annual checkup was only two days away, but a wave of panic washed over me, and I instinctively texted JJ.

"Pete can't die. I need him!"

I was overemotional and overreacting. Still stuck on high alert, I was exhausted and not thinking clearly. So I lifted him up onto our bed and lay down beside him, petting him for a while. That seemed to help us both.

A few hours later, I was standing at the kitchen sink when I saw him spontaneously lose his balance. He staggered sideways as if he were drunk, and the side of his little body rebounded harshly off the leg of a chair.

I dashed over to him, falling to my knees at his side.

Pete had always tried to hide when he was sick, and this time was no different. It made me sad that dogs always did that; I wished I could explain he'd never be in any trouble and that I just wanted to comfort him. But while he tried to scamper away this time, I watched him fall clumsily to the floor and vomit up a beige, watery pulp, unlike any dog puke I'd ever seen before.

I stared down at him in shock. This was unlike any sickness I'd ever seen. I'd never seen him, or any dog for that matter, ever collapse like that. I watched in horror as he struggled to get up—trying weakly but unable to—he slumped back down on the carpet in front of me once more.

Panic rushed through me and instinct took over. I didn't hesitate a second to scoop him up into my arms, repeating, "It's okay, it's okay," over and over as I ran straight for my car and laid him on his side in the backseat.

The position instantly looked unnatural to me, though maybe what was unnatural was that he wasn't reacting. There was vomit all over his sweet face, and he wasn't moving.

I drove as fast as I could while simultaneously calling the veterinarian, letting them know we were on our way. It was an eight-minute frantic car ride and, for that entire time, I kept glancing in the backseat at my baby, asking him to hold on.

"Hang on, Buddy. It's okay. It's going to be okay. I'm getting you help." A constant monologue of reassurance rolled out of my mouth.

I was in total shock. Consumed with fear and completely unaware of my physical surroundings, I careened into the parking lot, threw the car in park, and tore into the vet clinic clutching Pete. I barely even noticed the people in the waiting room, I just raced to the front of the line, thrusting my baby out to the reception desk and begging for help.

The vet hastily stepped out from around the corner, relieving the alarmed receptionist and reaching to take Pete's limp body from my outstretched arms. Someone else ushered me away, into a private exam room and away from curious, prying eyes.

I waited forever in that room alone, with only my giant fears. I wished I could call Marty, and I cried that I was alone. I cried for Pete.

Eventually, enough time passed that I stopped crying for a while. I fiddled with my phone and cursed the poor reception. I missed a call from our realtor and then listened to their voicemail; the contract on our house sale had fallen through, but I didn't even care. I prayed for my Petey to be alright. And then I cried and cried some more.

At one point, I got up and used the restroom, noticing for the first time that I was still wearing my Costco slippers. I called my dad from out in the lobby and cried a bit there, too.

When a vet finally came to speak to me, asking for my permission to run some tests, I was appalled by her question—confused as to why she would waste the time to ask something so obvious. "Do whatever you need to do," I told her. "Whatever it takes."

I waited by myself again and cried some more. Time ticked by.

A different vet came in next. "He's really sick," he told me, and a million thoughts raced through my head. Confusion and fear and frustration all twisted up inside of me.

It didn't make any sense; I needed to see him. I needed to see for myself what was going on.

At my insistence, the vet led me to the back of the clinic, and as we walked through swinging steel doors into a giant sterile room, I finally got to see my baby. He was lying wrapped in a blanket on what looked like a large operating table. His eyes were closed, there was a line of oxygen going to his little nose, and he was not moving.

I froze—unable to understand what I was seeing or how this had happened. Pete had been fine just that afternoon.

I felt someone trying to guide me forward, and a chair was rolled in front of me. I sat in it automatically. Leaning in carefully toward Pete's immobile body, I rested my arm on the table alongside the back of him, cradling his small frame to gently hug him toward me. My hand cupping the crown of his head.

Immediately in response to my presence, Pete roused. He opened his sweet eyes and looked directly at me—looked directly into my heart, my soul, and he nuzzled into me.

My heart broke. His reaction was so sweet I barely heard the nurse's breath catch as she watched us. I just held my baby close and nuzzled back into him.

He knew me.

Things were bad, and he was obviously sick, but he had communi cated in that moment that he still knew who I was, and I could sense that he wanted me close. Grief and regret hit me all at once. I should have asked to come sit with him sooner. "Is he on some kind of medication? What's happening? Why is he so drowsy?"

There was an awkward pause as the vet and the nurse looked at each other. "No," the vet replied. "He isn't on any medication."

I couldn't understand why he was so still—I demanded answers. A tumor on his spleen had potentially ruptured—I demanded they call a surgeon. There was no guarantee that surgery could save him—I said we had to try something. Anything. Money was no object; it was clear my baby was dying.

At my consent, the vet sprung into action. He unhooked the oxygen and carried my Petey, still wrapped in a blanket, out of the room, through the waiting room with all the prying eyes, and out to my car. I followed on his heels, watching as he laid Pete in the passenger seat. I rushed into the driver's side on reflex, still not understanding what was happening.

It wasn't until the vet started giving me directions to a *different* animal hospital that the realization hit.

I was supposed to do this alone.

A flood of panicked questions swirled through my mind. Yet oblivious to this, the vet just looked me square in the eye as he told me with equal parts compassion and authority to "drive safe." Then he shut the passenger door firmly, locking Pete and me inside.

We were alone.

I drove as fast as I dared, but we'd only made it a mile or two down the road when I could tell Pete wanted to be on my lap. He'd always loved car rides and chose to sit up front with me—and this time was no different.

He lifted his head weakly to look at me from the passenger seat, and I could tell he was struggling, barely able to hold his little head up on his own. I watched as he had to lean it awkwardly on the side of the console for support; it was such an unnatural angle. He wheezed at the effort, continuing to stare at me intently, still with a bit of that beige vomit around his mouth.

My heart clenched. "No, Buddy. It's hard for you to breathe like that." I reached over, cupped his chin in my hand, and helped him rest his little head back down onto the passenger seat. It killed me to see him like that. Killed me to have him sitting there alone.

Immediately, he lifted his head again—looking at me pleadingly, communicating to me with that single look—and I understood.

Racing down Highway 105, I reached over with my right arm curled and lifted his body up, lying him gently across my lap. Then I switched driving hands so I could tuck my left arm around him in support while I continued to drive way too fast. I cried, whimpering my reassurances.

He was silent and unmoving in my arms as I made the turn onto the 336 loop. I wasn't sure if he could hear me, yet I continued speaking to him anyway through my steady stream of tears. "It's okay. It's going to be okay. I love you."

He was so still that I wasn't sure if he was even alive, and I suspected, I feared, that he might be passing. I was holding him—my eyes were on the road, but my heart and my mind were entirely focused on him—I could no longer feel him breathing.

I sobbed as I choked out my final words to him: "It's okay. You can go." The words had fallen out of me unexpectedly, a flash from my memory, the same words I'd been told that my family had offered Kristin in her final hours. I didn't mean them—not really. Nothing about this was okay; I just didn't want him to suffer any longer, so I was trying to be brave. Trying to let him know I loved him and that this love would always greatly outweigh my own needs.

I pulled over at the first available opportunity, and as I put the car in park, I felt his last two breaths leave his body.

One big sigh. A long pause. A final exhale.

And then nothing.

I didn't move; I just sat there. I stared down at his little body in my arms, continuing to stroke him as the reality started to sink in. I had been there with him, for him, in his final moments. I had always been there for him, always been his mom, right until the end. And now he was gone.

I took only that moment for myself, and then, still in shock, I called the animal hospital we'd left only minutes prior.

"I think he died," I said through the sobs that threatened to take over. "How do I know for sure?"

Deep down, I already knew.

The vet directed me over the phone to gently touch the corner of his eye—Pete's beautiful, soulful green eyes. They were open but unmoving, and as I ever so gently brushed the corner of his eye with my fingertip, there was no reaction.

I put the car back in gear and started the drive back to the animal hospital. Much slower this time, with the dead body of my baby on my lap.

Back at the clinic, I struggled to lift Pete's body, limp and lifeless, and exit the car. He flopped, and his head lolled to one side—it wasn't right. It took me a minute or two to find a way to balance him, protect him, tuck him into the crook of my arm and my torso so that I could carry him inside.

I laid him on the exam table and asked the vet to test him again. "Please just make sure," I kept saying. But, of course, the vet was sure.

They gave me some time to sit with Pete, and I talked to him even though I knew he couldn't hear me. I petted him over and over, stroking his perfectly silky, soft vanilla fur. He was so beautiful, so perfect, even in death.

However, as I sat there with him, and time passed, I started to notice some things. His tongue, which had often poked out of his mouth so adorably in sleep, was visible now, too—but dry, frozen in place. And maybe only perceptible to me, but I thought it was grayer in color.

It wasn't right.

His eyes were frozen open but unseeing—and that wasn't right either. It didn't look like he was sleeping.

A rush of emotions flashed over me. Indignation. Disgust at how cruel life, and particularly the end of life, could be. Confusion and a small flash of horror. I couldn't understand the rush of any of these feelings through the tangle that was my grief.

On instinct, I stiffened my own posture, wanting to protect and defend his helpless little body. It didn't matter what his body was doing to him in death; this was not him. This was not who he had been in life. This was not my Pete.

I had to leave—abruptly sensing that I'd already been there too long. The animal hospital had maybe already closed while I'd been standing there in my sorrow. And I knew I didn't want to see Pete like that. I didn't want to have to watch his body change and stiffen and turn cold in front of me.

It was impossible to wrench myself away. I needed more time. Yet I knew in my heart that our time was over; this wasn't Pete anymore. My Petey was gone.

It was wrong to walk away, wrong to leave, but I took off his collar and forced myself to stand up.

The entire event had transpired over only a few hours, yet in that time, my life had been permanently altered. A part of me had died, too—when his heart had stopped beating, so had a piece of mine.

I'd felt more fear and panic that afternoon than I'd felt during the entire hurricane. More sadness and despair. And as I got into my car and drove home without him, I was gutted. More helpless, lost, and alone than ever.

Pete had been an unconditionally loving, supportive, and wholly non-judgmental witness to my life. He'd been a comfort to me through cities and countries moved, jobs changed, friends and family lost, health and illness—he'd been with me through it all.

The definition of a true friend.

And I'd known when I sat down with him at the operating table and he immediately nuzzled into me, and again when he wanted to climb onto my lap in the car one final time—that throughout his life, and in those final moments, he had loved me just as much as I had always loved him.

I had been his best friend, too.

PIECES

How did I get here?

How did I get to this place of complete physical and mental breakdown? How has this become my life?

The Lyme-guy continues to call this tick-borne illness, but I don't accept that. I don't deny I was bitten by a tick; what I struggle to understand is where and when I would have managed to contract the disease. The timeline of that one and only tick bite at six years old—versus the onset of illness thirty years later—doesn't stand to reason.

I stepped into some sort of nest when I was thirteen years old, out at Buffalo Pound Lake with my eighth-grade classmates. I forgot about that until recently, the itchy sensation while I hiked through the tall grasses up along the ridge on one of the hills. I scratched at my stomach and back absentmindedly until I became frustrated, lifting my navy T-shirt to find that my entire stomach was crawling with little brownish-black bugs.

My friends instantly started swatting at me. They flicked the bugs from my stomach and my back as I rolled down the waistband of my brown corduroy pants to expose another thick line of them. My ankles, my legs, my torso—all covered in hundreds and hundreds of ticks.

But I was okay; I was certain that none of them had bitten me. Later that night in my tent, I did a thorough tick check again and found no bites.

Not that it really matters, as the timeline of that incident isn't right either.

And I've been bitten by many things throughout my life—mosquitos, flies, wasps, and the like. I was constantly covered in bug bites during those summers I worked at the Burrowing Owl Centre. I've even been bitten by owls, a few cats, an angry Rottweiler, a temperamental duck. And one time, after vacationing at Deep Creek Lake in Maryland, we all came home with fleas.

Is any of that so unusual? Haven't we all been bitten by a multitude of things?

My family, perhaps still convinced that Lyme disease is only an "East Coast problem," reminds me that I lived in both New York and in Pennsylvania. Our blue house was only a few hours from Lyme, Connecticut, where the first US cases of the disease were discovered. It's hard to ignore a fact as ominous as that. Yet I don't recall a single tick bite during my time in the Northeast, and the timeline still isn't right.

I've even considered Texas and its lone star ticks, as well as the Rocky Mountain wood tick, too, as I have lived in those places more recently. But the reality is that every place I've ever lived and hiked has probably had some type of tick, whether I saw them or not. And the only bite I ever incurred happened when I was just six years old—yet I'd had a normal childhood. Perfect, in fact.

Throughout my entire life, absolutely no one would have ever described me as sick.

I may have been bitten, but my hesitation, distrust, and overall nonacceptance have always stemmed from the fear that *that* might not be my issue—or my only issue—and that we are treating the wrong thing. Because, at this point, I feel like we've really tested the Lyme-guy's theory. I've endured over a year's worth of his specialized treatments, and I'm *still* not any better.

What if I'm one of the few unaffected by their tick bite? Unaffected by tick-borne infection even? And the cause of my current problems is something entirely different?

What if I have something else?

Maybe these are the ramblings of a paranoid mind, isolated at home and trapped in bed. Or maybe it's the medical distrust I inherited from my father. Either way, I still believe these questions are fairly warranted, considering the treatment hasn't helped. And I think most of society would probably tend to agree; most of society remains distrustful that chronic Lyme is even real.

It is an unbelievable story to think that someone who's always identified as healthy has been fighting an illness for thirty-one years. To think that the bite from a single tick could've caused all of this. That one little bite could've so thoroughly destroyed a good life.

I'm not sure how anyone would be able to accept that.

Even if it is what the Lyme-guy thinks.

They say stress is immunosuppressive; it can activate a latent disease, trigger a relapse, or derail a treatment. Yet I wasn't stressed when I got sick. I flew out to Hawaii at the healthiest, most relaxed I'd been in years, so I struggle to see how that theory might apply. Not that it would confirm what disease I have, anyway.

I've got to think that there's more at play here, but my friends and family remain quick to blame those physical stressors: a drastic change in altitude, exposure to mold, injuries, medications, exercise, and diet. I don't get it. Not really. Although there is a small part of me that can get behind their logic—that a physical change could cause some physical symptoms—I suppose I do understand that. But could it really be that simple? Because now, following that logic, I can't help but wonder if maybe all along I shouldn't have been so quick to discount my emotional stressors, too: relocations, traumas, and grief.

I thought I was handling it; that's how I've always lived my life. Haven't I always just handled it? Yet when I think about it—I mean really think about it—maybe I wasn't "stressed" by my definition of the word, but those major life changes *are* a kind of stressor, too.

Maybe it was all of it combined.

In the "pot boiling over" theory, your health is seen as a big soup pot. When you're young, you only have in that pot a few genetic predispositions. Then, throughout your life, you accumulate some nutritional insufficiencies. Maybe some allergies. Hormonal imbalances, stresses, and traumas. These burdens on your health all slowly amass in the pot. You may even inadvertently collect some environmental pollutants, toxins, viruses, or infections. The load on your health may become perilously close to the top until, eventually, even the addition of a single stressor is enough to cause your health to spill over the edge.

It's not one single thing.

It's the cumulative effect of it all.

Others describe your health as a big red balloon that, when working correctly, bounces along happily in the world. Life events may put some pressure on it; it may get leaned on or squeezed. Sometimes, it's even going to fall. But again, when working correctly, your balloon is always supposed to bounce right back up.

I've got to wonder if *my* balloon could have already been under a fairly heavy pressure—squeezing it persistently, chronically. I've certainly been exposed to plenty of physical stressors, but I suppose I've also been burying my sensitivity, succumbing to people-pleasing and perfectionism, and internalizing my stress.

My soup pot might have been getting pretty full—because I started to fall apart as soon as I arrived in Colorado.

And while on our picture-perfect anniversary trip to Maui in the fall of 2019, my big red balloon finally popped.

My pot completely boiled over.

DENVER

THIRTY-FOUR YEARS OLD

It was only four days after Pete died, in the fall of 2017, that we moved to Colorado.

Between our busy work schedules, the tight timeline, and the flights in and out of IAH getting grounded due to the hurricane, we hadn't had a chance to fly up to see Denver in advance—or find ourselves a home. I'd had to sign a last-minute contract to secure an apartment, sight unseen, when I'd never even lived in an apartment before. Nor had I ever been to Denver. And despite my previous planning, we lost our professional movers as they assisted in the aftermath of Hurricane Harvey, leaving us to move the contents of an entire five-thousand-square-foot house on our own.

All aspects of that move felt like a disaster.

Although maybe it was just me, at the center of it all, that was the disaster.

We didn't have a going away party like I'd wanted. Devastated as I was after Pete's death, I didn't even make an effort to say goodbye to most of our friends or even our favorite neighbors. Instead, I sold as much of our furniture as I could online, and I hid alone in the house, numbly packing our belongings. I didn't eat, couldn't sleep, and I took a steady dose of antiemetic pills to keep myself from being physically sick.

Those four days passed in a blur.

A few of our closest friends came by in our final hours, arriving with smiles, mimosas, and food to share. Ashley helped me wrap all of my artwork, and Karla packed the garage, while the boys loaded the twenty-six-foot Penske truck that we'd had to rent last minute. And then I methodically walked through every single room of our empty lake house with Nicole and Christie, checking to make sure that nothing was left behind. My final moments with my closest friends, but I couldn't even enjoy them. Numb and overwhelmed with grief, I was devastated without my Petey there.

It took us an entire day to drive across the state of Texas. From the uncomfortable seats of the rented truck, I sent my parents a goofy selfie along the way—an attempt at some sort of reassurance, evidence that I was doing all right. Even though I wasn't.

I couldn't stop playing back Pete's death in my mind, worrying about how he had felt in that final hour. I prayed it had been okay for him—that he had sensed every ounce of my love as I had held him, spoken to him, and wept while he'd passed in my arms. His death had left me tormented, unable to wrap my head around what actually happens to someone when they die.

On a basic level, I understood that he was gone, but I struggled to know what that meant exactly. Where was "gone" precisely? Was it an actual place, or did we simply someday cease to exist? My questions were intrusive and ruminating. I couldn't get my mind to stop.

I felt like I'd failed him somehow. Failed to keep him with me, keep him safe, keep him alive. It seemed a part of me would forever feel responsible for him, and I couldn't handle not knowing where he had gone and if he was okay. I could barely bring myself to look in the empty backseat or down at my empty lap.

I was hyperaware of his absence in the truck.

But also, just hyperaware of his absence.

A hollowness consumed me. An emptiness, a suffocating incompleteness. I was overcome with a sense of having lost something or left something behind, and with every mile we drove away from Texas, my panic rose.

I *had* left something behind.

I'd left him.

As a child in the '80s, I'd had one of those brightly colored rubber bouncy balls—a hard, dense little thing that rebounded crazy high. I used to sneak into my mother's large and beautifully affixed bathroom with that ball, shutting the door quietly behind me. Then I'd throw that thing as hard as I could into the large jetted soaker tub, aiming for the side wall. And I'd watch that neon rocket ricochet and zing, zooming off the ivory, hammering back and forth before it finally escaped the confines of the tub and bounced freely off the bathroom walls, the ceiling, and the floor. All the while, I stood in the center of it, dodging out of the way as it flew erratically all around me.

It was chaos.

And *that* is how my grief felt.

Uncontrollable. Untamed. Unpredictable. Pinballing all over the place, between the stages of grief in no predictable order, as I stood helplessly at the center of it all.

We were moving, and I was bringing everything with me except a large piece of my heart—a large piece of my family. We were two now, not three; in the history of all our moves, this was the first one without our Pete. So we sat in silence; Marty drove solemnly while I cried steadily beside him for the second day in a row on the road. Mile after mile, and hour after hour.

Once in Denver, it didn't take long for me to notice that I couldn't breathe. The air was incredibly dry, especially compared to Houston, and with the high altitude, there wasn't enough oxygen. I couldn't walk or climb stairs, let alone exercise. I was short of breath while trying to speak or eat dinner, and even while lying in bed at night.

I was told that everyone experienced this when they first moved to such a high altitude, but it didn't improve within a week for me, or even a month, like people had said. I got a humidifier, shoved some petroleum jelly up my nostrils to prevent nosebleeds, and I found a new doctor—doctor-number-one in Denver—who prescribed me a rescue inhaler for what we could only assume was the return of my childhood asthma.

I started having abdominal pain, sharp and constant, in my lower right quadrant. I went back to that same clinic, where doctor-number-two dismissed my concerns, telling me that I must have pulled a muscle while moving. It did sound like valid reasoning; though it didn't explain why my feet hurt like the bones had broken overnight. The surface level of the skin was painful to the touch, and my heels were numb and tingling. I had pain that moved around, terrible insomnia, what I thought was sciatica, and again, what I thought was piriformis syndrome. But doctor-number-two only looked at me dubiously and suggested I get insoles.

So I did—and I dove into work, trying to forget it all. I was in the process of designing and constructing a twenty-thousand-square-foot office for Marty's new company, as well as a new modern home for us. I tried to keep my focus on that.

I couldn't wait to get out of the small apartment. Marty was living part-time in North Dakota, setting up a field office for the new company, and with all of our meaningful possessions still in storage, I lived by myself in that undecorated unit. Our mattress was thrown on the floor, and I used boxes for make-shift nightstands. Worse yet, it was a unit that had been selected with Pete in mind (the contract signed only days before his unexpected death). It was ground-level, with direct access to a common area where people and dogs regularly socialized, and the view of *that* out the windows was brutal. It was a constant daily reminder that our Pete wasn't there.

I was used to Marty traveling for work, but now it was different. Pete had always been my constant. Regardless of Marty's travel schedule, regardless of what state or country we lived in, Pete had always been my sense of security—my familiarity, my stability, and my sense of home. I was lost without him.

I kept all of the blinds closed so I wouldn't have to see any of the dogs outside, but the small, dark apartment became more like a prison cell as the months dragged on. There was no part of Denver that was starting to feel like home for me; without my boys, I was completely alone in my new city and state.

I needed out. No matter how much I tried to focus on my work, my passion for design—CAD software always open on my screen, papers strewn about, my tape measure and architect's ruler always in use—none of it was enough to distract me. I still cried all the time.

I spent most of my nights wandering the small apartment with insomnia, choking back sobs. While during the days, I was hit with flashbacks of my last week in Texas, erupting into tears in the car, at lunch, or even in the aisles of TJ Maxx. I became desperate to avoid any mementos, photos, songs, or certain pieces of clothing. I even stopped keeping in touch with some of my friends in Texas simply because I couldn't bear the reminder.

It felt strange that I hadn't said a proper goodbye, and even stranger that the last time I'd seen some of them was soaking wet in the midst of a hurricane. I wanted to block all of those memories from my mind. Forget Texas ever existed. Yet Charlene had her employees calling and texting me incessantly.

Everything with Charlene was still a "911." It wasn't anything with my designs or clients, thankfully, but it was administrative things that they called me about. It was evident they were struggling to run the office without me. I got texts, phone calls, and fifteen-minute rambling frantic voicemails. They wanted to fire Camila. They couldn't find Jessica's phone number. They didn't know how to place custom orders through Leigh.

No one ever asked how I was doing during these calls, and it felt like I'd never left—that I was still somehow beholden to Charlene's tyranny. While through all this, the woman who'd bought our lake house wouldn't stop texting me either.

"What type of light bulbs are in the dining room chandelier?"

"What kind of tile is around the pool?"

"Where would I buy those?"

"Who built the pool?"

"Can you send a link for that?"

I politely answered all of Karen's questions initially, reminding her that I'd left all of that information in an organized binder on the kitchen island. But she kept bombarding me, repeating many of the same questions I'd already answered.

"What dentist did you use here?"

"Where's a good place to eat?"

"Who built the pool? I want to talk to them about what kind of tile this is. Do you know what kind of tile this is?"

"What's the pool guy's name again?"

"Who built the pool?"

"What's his name?"

"What did you say this tile was called?"

Her texts were constant reminders of the home that Marty and I had shared with Pete. The home that Pete had collapsed in. The home that I'd had to return to alone after he'd died in my arms. I finally ignored Karen; it was out of character for me, and it went against my people-pleasing tendencies, yet I knew it had to be done. Ignoring her may have caused me some angst, but her questions were causing more.

Then, our realtor from Texas emailed us, outright and inappropriately, asking us for thousands of dollars because Karen had decided she wanted new windows. It didn't make any sense. The house was only two years old and had no defects. I had personally ensured that the warranty work had been diligently completed before I'd sold it, including having all of those windows inspected by the manufacturer. Yet his email was laced with accusations and threats that we, "as good people," should be paying for Karen's new windows.

I'd never liked him. Mr. Larch had attempted to represent both us as the sellers and Karen as the buyer in the transaction—a clear conflict of interest right from the start. I felt he'd behaved inappropriately the entire time, so I shouldn't have been surprised by his email—but I was upset by his timing.

He'd sent it on Christmas Eve and given me another reason to cry. I ended up ignoring him, too.

That's when the decorator at Charlene's office contacted me.

"Hey, so I'm standing here," Mark said as a way of greeting when I answered the phone.

"What's up?" I pictured him standing in one of Charlene's dreary-looking offices. Fabric samples strewn about on the desk in front of him.

"What color are these walls?"

His question took me by surprise. My mind conjured the warm beige of the office interior I knew would be surrounding him. Sherwin-Williams Kilim perhaps, though I didn't know for sure; it had been painted long before I'd ever joined the firm.

"Sea Salt?"

I froze—and my heart did a little flip. "Pardon?" I asked slowly, even though instinctually, I already knew. There was only one place I'd ever used that paint color; in my entire career, I'd only ever used it once. I'd saved it. All of that time, I'd saved it. Just for me.

"I'm in your house!" Mark exclaimed joyfully.

I had to sit down, collapsing into one of only two chairs we had in the apartment. How could this be? Mark had never been to my lake house before, we hardly knew each other. What was he talking about? How was he even there? Why was he there? There could only be one possible explanation, and my brain answered my own rapid-fire questions just as he voiced it aloud.

"I'm going to redesign it!"

I could practically see him clapping his hands together as he jumped up and down in our elegant great room. The crystal orb chandelier sparkling above him. The infinity pool and the lake visible through the grand wall of windows behind.

He was going to work for the woman who had purchased our lake house. The woman who wouldn't stop texting me questions about lightbulbs and pool tile. The woman who was asking for thousands of dollars to replace perfectly good windows. Mark was going to be working for Karen. Mark was going to redesign *my* lake house—the house that I'd spent nearly two years perfecting—and he wasn't even a real designer.

In a daze, I told him something vague, like, "That's great," and I let him drone on until I felt I'd fulfilled whatever social niceties were required of me in that situation. Then I told him that I, too, had to get back to work, and we hung up. The whole time, I couldn't stop picturing him painting over my perfect Sea Salt walls and tearing apart the picture-perfect memories I had with Marty and Pete in that house. It was all too much.

I ended up ignoring Mark's subsequent calls and texts, along with Charlene's, Karen's, and Mr. Larch's, too. And just when I thought it couldn't get any weirder, I received a string of very confusing late-night texts from my most favorite client back in Texas.

I had worked with Mr. and Mrs. Moore intensely for over a year on their multi-million-dollar custom home. I'd made every selection for their construction, as well as for the furniture and decor, and I'd gotten to know them personally while the three of us had hung every single one of their family photos to complete each space.

They were down-to-earth and sweet, an older couple with an adorable relationship that had at first reminded me of my parents. We'd gotten along quite well, and their project had been one of my favorites, but her words in those late-night texts jumped off the screen at me.

"Your sick scam sucked me in."

"Such a sexy risqué moment for the two of you."

"Maybe you, as a professional businesswoman, should not be leaching after older, rich men clients. Is this the reason you were fired from Charlene's? Be honest."

"I pray you have found a better place to do business and not CHEAT your clients in more ways than one."

"If I can prevent you from ever treating another customer that way, believe God, it will be done."

Her words made me sick. The accusation of an affair might have been the most hurtful thing anyone had ever said to me. I was appalled, horrified, even. Her husband was old—gross, old. Beyond that, I'd never even been alone in a room with her husband; I'd always met with them together as a couple. It had been one of the reasons I'd liked them so much. Seeing their love and support of one another as they'd attended every meeting and made every decision together, Mr. and Mrs.

Moore had appeared to be a true partnership. I was devastated, both by the realization that their marriage wasn't as idyllic as I'd thought, but also that her accusation might now be tarnishing my reputation in Texas when I wasn't even there to defend it.

I was humiliated. Yet JJ and Marty both howled with laughter when I told them, unable to imagine a more preposterous accusation. I hadn't been fired—I hadn't been fired from anything in my entire life. And no amount of money would ever be a motivator for me, not only did we have plenty of our own, I was in *love* with my husband.

I crafted a reply with JJ and Marty's help, but I didn't wait to see if Mrs. Moore would answer. I promptly deleted and blocked her contact info on my phone.

It had simply been too much, all at once.

Some of my friends and family members worried that I was exhibiting signs of post-traumatic stress disorder, yet I refused to consider the notion. All of my beautiful memories and experiences in Texas had slowly been tarnished, and I was grieving—maybe I even had some dysthymia, a low-level persistent depression. But I thought using words like trauma or labels like PTSD was being overly dramatic.

I kept my focus looking forward, and I did everything I could for my health. I restricted my diet even further by going vegan, ceased all pharmaceuticals, distracted myself with work (clinging to the belief that our new modern home would be better than our lake house had ever been), and I fell in love with yoga, practicing it daily.

It was low impact and felt kind to my body. It felt therapeutic. There was a sense of connection each time I stepped on my mat. A connection to myself: my body, movement, and breath. My mind, my heart, and my soul. A connection to others, a sense of community and belonging—though a connection to something even bigger as well. I somehow felt connected to the world outside of the studio, to nature, to the universe, and even to a higher power.

I practiced with my eyes closed and occasionally found that through my movement and breath, unbeknownst to me, tears had been falling onto my mat. I took this to mean that my heart, my grief, and my mind were healing when I practiced yoga.

But as I rolled up my mat each day and made my way out of the studio, all of my pains came rushing back.

Nothing felt right.

Fifteen months into my time in Denver, I started to suspect my friends and family had been correct all along. My reaction no longer seemed normal—my soul felt broken. I didn't think the gaping hole in my heart would ever heal. And my body wasn't right either.

None of my issues had gone away. I still had the insomnia, the persistent pains, the numbness, and the shortness of breath. But I'd been accumulating even more ailments, too—progressively worsening, despite how hard I kept trying to heal myself through kindness and nutrition, as I'd always done before.

Doctors one, two, and three at my new clinic in Denver all continued to dismiss me, assuring me that I was "fine," yet I knew instinctively that I wasn't. Grief couldn't possibly be the cause of this, and it certainly wasn't stress. I could no longer ignore the nagging sense of unease.

When my current design jobs wrapped up in January of 2019, I spontaneously took some time off of work. Pausing for the first time in my adult life, I said no to all incoming requests.

I'd never said *no* before. Not only was it completely out of character for me, I hadn't even planned to do it. I declined several residential design jobs, a restaurant renovation, and a luxury Paul Mitchell salon, all in that first month. I didn't really explain myself, and I didn't even have a plan. But somehow, I knew I needed to focus on my health. I needed to hit pause. I needed a break.

For the next nine months, I did everything right. I slept well and relaxed, ate healthy, and exercised lightly. And I was thrilled to be planning a vacation to Maui for our upcoming anniversary in October.

I wanted to walk the beach, snorkel, and swim with the sea turtles; I'd even read that there were a few areas where we might be able to see wild dolphins. I'd planned some epic hikes for us as well, reading all the adventure blogs I could in advance of the trip. I wanted to climb mountains and volcanoes and explore the depths of the jungle—use ropes to scale the slippery slopes, cliff dive, and swim in natural waterfalls. Hawaii sounded to me like an adventurer's dream.

Instead, my life fell completely apart on that picture-perfect vacation; right there in Hawaii, an unexplained cardiac event brought my life to a grinding halt.

It was as if my body was saying, "Thank you for this break. I need to let you know what's been going on with me." And then it did. I'd become ill by the same description that Hemingway once wrote: gradually and then suddenly. The underlying cause may have been insidious, but when the illness finally struck, it was neither gradual nor subtle. There wasn't anything mild or ambiguous about my situation.

I was in crisis mode.

My poised facade came crumbling down, and my laid-back nature and permanent easy smile vanished. My once perfectly maintained household fell apart. My decline happened fast, and the lesson learned was equally so. For once in my adult life, I learned to ask for help.

I pleaded for help, actually, as I told my story repeatedly to doctors one, two, and three, as well as doctor-number-four, my new cardiologist. I had bloodwork taken, often upward of thirty vials drawn in a single day. Respiratory and cardiac tests. Ultrasounds, X-rays, EKGs, and CT scans. Yet the only thing anyone could find was that my thyroid and cholesterol were slightly off but still within the normal range; my vitamin D was low, even though I lived in one of the sunniest places in America; and my stomach pain was assumed to be endometriosis, which doctor-number-three claimed would be hard to prove but easily solved by simply removing my uterus.

"You're not planning to have kids anyway, right?"

I'm only thirty-six, I thought, as my heart sank at her dismissiveness. Though I was too meek to say it aloud.

My teeth started searing in fiery pain six weeks later on Thanksgiving weekend, and I suffered through both facial and chest electrocutions daily after that. A few weeks later, in January 2020, I awoke to a dislocated jaw.

I started seeing bugs. My left eye was fine, but in my right eye, there was movement—a sudden onset of severe floaters that resembled worms, blobs, or even sperm floated across my field of vision. I developed a persistent dry cough in addition to the shortness of breath. An acne-like rash and dark circles appeared under my eyes, and I could no longer sufficiently regulate my body temperature.

I pursued more doctors, dentists, and surgeons, yet my symptoms only continued to pile up. My hair fell out in chunks, disgusting maybe, but mostly it scared me. I tried three more doctors. And then two more. I cried while doctor-number-nine couldn't even bring himself to look me in the eye as he shrugged and left the exam room.

COVID hit in March 2020, leaving me to research on my own. My Google searches kept coming up with inflammation (it seemed to be at the root of all disease), though I couldn't figure out why. When finally, on May 8, 2020, at the height of the pandemic, I saw a post on Instagram titled "20 Root Causes of Chronic Inflammation." I immediately forwarded the list to JJ and Marty.

The three of us scoured that list for clues. Clinging to it like it would be the treasure map back to my elusive health, we spent the night researching and considering every single item on that list. Armed with a new direction, the two of them contacted a few more new doctors on my behalf. JJ found me a new naturopath, and Marty found a Lyme-guy —an integrative, functional medicine doctor who specialized in Lyme.

Dr. Ryan wasn't warm; although it was during COVID and Marty and I were meeting with him over telemedicine, so I took that into consideration. But he didn't even flinch or express compassion when I confessed what I thought were some truly horrific symptoms. Instead, he stayed detached. Calm and factual. He bordered on cold and even a little socially awkward. He wasn't my cup of tea at all.

He looked to be about Marty's age, not quite forty. Tall and thin. His round tortoise glasses somehow exuded both trendy and nerdy at the same time. And his hair, while at one point might've been professionally cut, appeared disheveled and a bit overgrown. He wore a plain, colored dress shirt with no white coat or stethoscope around his neck.

The overall look, likely intended to appear businesslike, had a bit of laid-back vibe instead. An I-don't-care vibe. Or maybe just an I'm-bad-at-details kind of vibe. Which, combined with his dark and broody expressionless demeanor, made him seem a bit cooler than he probably was.

His office in the background didn't look like a typical medical office either, which only added to the intimidation. He sat at a desk (that part was fine), but there was what looked to be a chiropractor's table off to one side when I was certain this man was not a chiropractor. On his right, a library of strange-looking cassettes and vials was lined up along the otherwise barren wall. There were no photographs, no personal effects, only a handful of framed degrees and certifications hung to his left. It was a fairly minimalist space; it didn't give anything away.

I didn't trust it. And I wasn't sure if I trusted him.

Yet as Marty and I sat at our kitchen island, with Dr. Ryan on the screen in front of us, I noticed he wasn't trying to sell us on anything—himself, his clinic, pricey supplements, or additional alternative treatments and tests. He didn't even try to sell us on his success rate.

He was honest. He told us it was going to be a marathon, and that there was no cure or guarantee. He wasn't flashy about it, and he made no promises. He was the exact opposite of the charlatans my suspicious and paranoid mind had conjured and feared.

If this was his sales pitch, it really wasn't very good.

Dr. Ryan said very little in that first meeting. He did not try to dismiss or normalize anything Marty said; rather, he listened for the entire hour. He listened to every single crazy and disconnected symptom, and not once did he interrupt—I wasn't used to that type of attention. By the end, my face was red with embarrassment. I was certain this doctor (barely older than I was, tall, dark, and almost handsome) was going to laugh at me.

Instead, through the screen, I saw him look me square in the eye as he said in a monotone: "I think you have Lyme disease."

My life was forever changed by those six words.

I'd never considered Lyme before that week. It hadn't once come up on any of our internet searches, and he'd been the first doctor, after nine other doctors, to mention it, let alone suggest I be tested.

He'd referred us to specialty labs we'd never heard of, IgeneX and DNA ConneXions, so we dove into research yet again, and I read my first few articles and descriptions of Lyme later that night.

For the first time in all of my years of research, I sensed an immediate likeness.

I got myself tested the following week using a provoked method. This meant that after taking a few days of antibiotics to stir up any hiding infections, I used a far-infrared sauna and ran up and down my street to release a suspected *Borrelia* from where it might be hiding. Then I waited an hour for any of these potentially released microbes to make their way into my urinary tract, finally peeing in the sample cup to be sent away for testing.

It sounded like complete nonsense—but I did do it, as Dr. Ryan had sworn it would be accurate. And a week later, I received a diagnosis.

Late-stage neurological Lyme disease.

It was found all throughout my body; the infection, the attack, was multi-systemic. It flowed throughout my body in my lymph, as well as in my blood. It was in my muscles and my joints and my organs: heart, liver, kidneys, bladder, and spleen. It was even in my brain.

I had a total of five active live infections, five diseases, all of which were believed to have been passed to me from the bite of a single tick. I had two different types of *Borrelia* bacteria—*Borrelia burgdorferi* and *Borrelia recurrentis*—also known as Lyme disease and tick-borne relapsing fever. I had two different strains of *Babesia*—*Babesia divergens* and *Babesia duncani*—meaning two different types of babesiosis, a parasitic and hemolytic disease caused by microscopic malaria-like parasites. And lastly, I had an intracellular parasite called *Bartonella henselae*—bartonellosis—colloquially known as cat scratch disease, though apparently commonly vector-borne as well. And each one of these co-infections was increasing the severity of the other, complicating my prognosis.

Sitting on the edge of my bed, I stared, stunned at the results in my email—the official black and white words on the screen staring ominously back. I knew I needed to text Marty to ask him to come up from the basement. I had to text JJ. I had to tell them both that the results had arrived. Instead, I sat there motionless, unsure what I'd even tell them.

The moment felt monumental. Surreal. Every symptom was now explained, and a giddy, nervous energy overtook me. I was relieved I wasn't crazy. I felt vindicated, my fears validated. I wanted to call all of the doctors and dentists who had not believed me. I *had* been right—this was all connected.

I thought I might start to laugh or even cry—yet oddly, I did neither. I just sat there, gaping at my screen.

It was the end of a very long and hard journey.

But also, I wondered if it might be the beginning of another.

Horror was starting to creep in. Denial was starting to take hold. Distrust in the specialty labs *and* in Dr. Ryan was settling in. What did we know about this Lyme-guy, anyway? What did we know about this disease? From what I'd heard, Lyme could be brutal and lifelong, and its treatment extremely dangerous. This couldn't be right.

I may have wanted an answer. A diagnosis.

But not this answer. Not this diagnosis.

UNACCEPTABLE

THIRTY-SIX YEARS OLD

Chronic Lyme disease.

With those words, everything changed.

I still sat there on my bed, unmoving, staring at the results in my hand. I couldn't believe it. Health had always been important to me, a priority. I ate healthy, and I was fit. My residual self-image, who I would have always described myself to be, was healthy.

But now that image, that identity, was being questioned. I was being told that not only was I *not* healthy—I'd never *been* healthy. In fact, I'd been nothing but a ticking time bomb.

As a straight-A student and a top athlete, my Lyme test was the first in my life I'd ever failed. And as someone who'd always valued control, I had unexpectedly encountered something that was completely beyond it.

Lyme couldn't possibly be right. It was more than a shock to me; it was a mystery that didn't make any sense.

I was lucky I'd been journaling over the years. Throughout a decade of unexplained symptoms and (mis)diagnoses, I'd accumulated quite a bit of information about myself—and my mom had unknowingly done a similar thing. Always one to prioritize her girls, she'd documented our lives both in scrapbooks and in journals; she, too, had amassed quite a bit of data.

I took that information and immediately started writing. I wasn't even sure where I was going with it initially, but I felt I had a lot to say and even more to figure out.

I looked back at my life, and even though my thoughts and memories would only come to me through the inflammation as random blips, I worked through the fog. With my family and with my doctors alike, I wrote everything down.

I had a zillion webpages open on my phone at all times, and just as many multi-colored Post-it notes strewn about my desk on which I'd hastily scribbled random words. Dark blue, light blue, mint green, and yellow. Scraps of white torn out of notebooks. I'd pinned notes to the wall and taped them to my desk—words and sentence fragments, things scratched out, and lists upon lists of symptoms.

Twenty-five symptoms.

Trepidatiously and without any better theories or options, I started a Lyme disease treatment. Weeks passed, and then months passed, when somehow, the summer was already over and those twenty-five symptoms had been replaced by thirty-seven.

I tried to understand. Learning everything I could, I read medical journals, blogs, books, and websites—taking notes and comparing my life to those of other mysteriously ill patients. I knew that in order to someday believe, trust, and keep moving forward, I had to first understand.

Fifty-six symptoms. That number was my wake-up call; we all have idiosyncrasies, and we all have ailments, but I knew *that* number was unacceptable. I bounced around between the stages of grief after that, yet my mysterious illness didn't care. Fall faded to winter, and as the year 2020 gave way to 2021, my list of symptoms only continued to grow.

Sixty-five symptoms.

Seventy symptoms.

Eighty-nine symptoms.

My time was running out; still, I continued to try and solve the mystery of my health with every ounce of strength that I had left. It was an impossible task, but I knew I had come to terms with my illness. For my own survival, I had to somehow learn to accept the unacceptable.

One hundred symptoms.

They were all layered, one on top of another. It was hard to tell where one symptom ended and another began, making it nearly impossible to define them, describe them, let alone list or rank them.

I spent a lot of time trying to make sense of that list of one hundred symptoms. I reorganized it and tried to control it, grouping like items into categories, thinking it could help explain them and make the list appear shorter. Yet each time a new symptom arose, I had to go back in and group more and more things together—convincing myself that it was just a different aspect of the previous symptom, anyway.

I forever tried to keep that list under one hundred. An arbitrary number perhaps, but still one I refused to surpass.

On many occasions, I considered deleting that list altogether—perhaps getting closer to believing a diagnosis as I knew normal, healthy people didn't have such long lists of symptoms to try and organize. But I didn't delete it. That list was something tangible, a fact that could not be argued or forgotten when my memory was impaired. I thought that list would be the most essential clue to my mystery.

What I didn't expect to find, however, was that the life stories I wrote would actually give me my biggest clue.

I'd initially written them for nostalgia and as a means of remembering my true self—thinking that if I was going to imminently die, there should be a record of who I once had been. I thought those life stories would highlight the dichotomy of how healthy, happy, and active my life had been prior to falling ill in Hawaii in 2019. What I hadn't expected to discover, was how intertwined the illness had actually been throughout my life. And I was forced to come to terms with the fact that maybe I did always have a few more symptoms than were typically normal. A few more symptoms than I was willing to admit. I acquiesced that maybe I wasn't as healthy as I'd previously thought.

It was with *that* realization that I started to believe in a diagnosis.

Through my own writing, I saw that my symptoms had all started in my youth. There were the nosebleeds and the "asthma," of course, but those alone wouldn't have been enough to convince me. It was the intense sickness that occurred during my first year of university at age eighteen: anxiety, tachycardia, a severe bout of mono, followed by hepatitis, jaundice, hair loss, shingles, shooting body pains, and another bout of mono. I could see *that* had most certainly not been normal.

I then saw the other episode that started in Pittsburgh, the one at age twenty-seven where anxiety escalated to agoraphobia, and I had my first major depressive episode. I was plagued by vertigo and brain zaps, neck and bladder issues, drenching night sweats, pain and numbness, all followed by diagnoses of perioral dermatitis, leaky gut, and celiac disease.

Finally, the third episode at age thirty-six in Hawaii is what proved irrefutably to me that something was horribly wrong.

I thought of the pot-boiling-over theory, and the big red balloon, and of the different diseases I'd read that could lie dormant and then flare when triggered by a stressor. Through my writing, I saw all of my episodes were definitely that.

Three episodes (at ages thirty-six, twenty-seven, and as early as eighteen) showed me that it had all started right there in Saskatchewan, long before I'd ever moved out East. A single tick bite as a small six-year-old child, no other explanation, as simple as that. The infection had been present in me all along.

Lyme.

It was, and had always been, Lyme disease.

It was all connected.

My life entangled with the illness had been a slow and convoluted spiral—episodes of extreme illness and moments of madness, intermixed with years of stability and accomplishment. Though as each episode increased in severity, as well as in length, the presentation changed and the edges became progressively more ill-defined, only adding to the confusion. It was nearly impossible to know where I ended and the disease began—how much of my life was normal ups and downs and how much of it had been the illness all along. The disease had been slowly taking over, silently and stealthily, until it eventually infiltrated every aspect of my life. And I saw it. After decades of chasing answers across two provinces and four states, I finally stopped questioning.

My Lyme-guy, Dr. Ryan, had been right all along.

It was unacceptable what Lyme had taken from me—settling a fog over me and making me question myself all those times. The reason for my anxiety and insecurity, the constant weight on my shoulders, the pit in my stomach, the reason for my hesitations. I wondered if maybe I could have done more, could have *been* more. I wondered who I would have been or how my life would have unfolded without that heavy burden of being unwell.

I thought a piece of my heart might always ache for the loss of what could have been—and that wasn't something that was countable in days.

My life had turned out so differently than I'd always imagined, and I knew going forward it would be different from the lives of those around me. There would be long-term consequences of the illness and its toxic treatment on my body.

It was unacceptable that I hadn't received a diagnosis sooner. For three decades, my doctors treated my unusual symptoms and ignored the bigger picture, and when things completely fell apart for me, I was dismissed. My voice was not heard.

TMJ issues are a common symptom of Lyme, yet not a single doctor, dentist, or TMJD "specialist" we spoke with ever made that connection. If there had been a diagnosis sooner, maybe the dislocation of my jaw could have been avoided altogether. I found *that* to be unacceptable, too.

The ambiguity and controversy surrounding Lyme were unacceptable, as was the fact that politics and profits had been getting in the way of helping patients in need. It was unacceptable to be denied disability or insurance coverage for treatment. Unacceptable that any person should be sent home to "handle" the potentially lethal symptoms of Lyme disease without any medical support.

It was unacceptable to not chew, smile, or speak for nearly two years (still with no end in sight). And unacceptable that anyone should have to black out daily.

The fear, confusion, and loss of self-confidence were unacceptable. The guilt, humiliation, and shame. Losing your mind and yourself. Favoring death over life. Explosions. Electrocutions. They were all completely unacceptable.

I was bit by a bug thirty-one years ago and nearly *died* because of it. But with time, I learned to accept it all.

THE END OF ONE CHAPTER

I folded into child's pose and cried into my mat.
And watched the documentary *Heal* on Netflix repeatedly.

I meditated.
I believed.
I prayed.
I wept.

I did yoga.
Far-infrared saunas.
And yoga *in* the far-infrared sauna.

I journaled.
Went to therapy.
And took neuroplasticity brain retraining courses.

I tried allopathic medicine.
Osteopathic medicine.
Alternative, functional, integrative, and naturopathic medicines.

I did everything the doctors prescribed.
And took everything the doctors prescribed.

Natural herbal painkillers.
CBD, cannabis, and curcuminoids.
Homeopathic painkillers.
Pharmaceutical painkillers.
Over-the-counter, prescription, and narcotics.

I tried alcohol to relax.
And then abstained to reduce inflammation.

Breathed purified air.
Drank reverse-osmosis water.
And followed an intentional anti-inflammatory diet.

I stepped way outside of my comfort zone.

Took a vow of silence.

And surrendered.

I lost hope.
And found hope.
Recommitting time and time again.

But with chronic illness, it is just that.

There is no end.

In the months following my epiphany of acceptance, unfortunately, not a lot changed. I mostly remained bedridden, living my nightmare in a silent and dark bubble. Every day, we considered at which point to return to the hospital.

I alternated between hope and optimism with each new test finding and new proposed treatment—and despair. I blamed myself that I still must be doing it wrong as we watched my body break down in ways that should have only been happening to someone twice my age. Osteoarthritis. Bulged and herniated discs. Bone spurs. Lesions. Bladder failures. Loss of nerve function. Loss of motor control. Loss of vision. Loss of memory.

So many, many losses.

It was a blur of painful symptoms and loneliness, seemingly useless medical tests, detox baths, and failed protocols. I threatened to quit treatment altogether on a monthly basis and weighed the option of death just as often.

At times, I was able to convince myself I didn't ever want to die and that I just wanted an escape. I wanted my current life situation to end—not my actual life. But at other times, I was unable to see a way out. The intrusive thoughts were inescapable, and the pull of the suicide was dangerous. Imminent.

I'd placate myself by saying I only had to stay alive until a specific date, and then I'd be allowed to go—getting myself through a few more desperate days with that sweet promise of relief. Then I'd somehow muster up the strength to pick a new date, a few more days out, surviving like that in three-day increments.

Vaccines became available for COVID in the spring of 2021, and the world finally started to open up.

As did my options.

I added treatments with a rife machine and photobiomodulation (red light, near-infrared light, and cold low-level laser therapy). I tried lymphatic massage, cupping, physical and craniosacral therapy. I dry skin brushed and attempted gua sha. I used castor oil packs on my abdomen, and then on my face, and then anywhere I was feeling pain. There was reflexology, acupressure, and acupuncture, and when those didn't help, I turned to chiropractic. And a variety of physical therapy devices were used to realign my neck, straighten my back, and stretch my intercostal muscles. I tried multiple neuroplasticity or brain retraining programs. I even purchased a mini vibrator for my jaw after watching the documentary *Introducing Selma Blair*.

I became obsessed with the idea that mold, EMFs, or altitude could be inhibiting my progress. I was tormented by the thought that we needed to move, that I'd never be able to heal in the same place where I'd fallen ill. Or maybe it was heavy metals or some emotional trauma from my past that I had yet to overcome (and couldn't even remember).

I researched fanatically, convinced I must have craniocervical instability or that a simple atlas adjustment was the solution. I read up on peptides and stem cells, hyperthermia, shamans, and more, compiling lists upon lists of ideas I would try next.

Information would be my salvation; my cure, I was certain, must lie somewhere under one of those stones yet unturned.

None of it worked. And when it became clear that none of those things were going to heal my dislocated jaw either, and there didn't seem to be anyone or any way to pop it back into place, I sought help from dentist-number-ten—a biological dentist named Dr. Kim.

I started wearing a neuromuscular TMJ splint at their recommendation—a maxillary anterior guided orthotic (MAGO). It was a thick, chunky plastic device that fit over my upper teeth like a mouthguard intended for tackle football, yet I had to wear it twenty-four hours a day. Its concept was to provide a safe, balanced environment for my jaw to rest while my brain reset, gradually reprogramming the muscles to heal my bilateral dislocations.

I made some progress with it, although it was minimal. The muscle spasms ceased, and I did gain a bit more control. I learned to speak and chew again, but this was only with the orthotic in place. In the end, I still remained in pain, with none of my teeth even coming close to occluding.

My jaw may have been doing better, but it was still quite far from actually being *better*.

I went in to have my wisdom teeth removed, along with cavitation surgery, as a last-ditch effort. A Hail Mary attempt to fix my bite. Yet even though I knew it was ridiculous and not the reason behind the dislocation, I couldn't help but be disappointed when I awoke to find that my remaining teeth still didn't touch.

I sought help from more doctors, more surgeons, and more alternative practitioners. And I tried more treatments, spending tens of thousands of dollars more. I dedicated all of my limited energy to my healing; I spent more time in bed and more time isolated as more opportunities passed me by.

More. More. More.

Still, I remained steadfast in my resolve to heal myself.

And month after month, we slowly pieced together more of the puzzle.

In addition to my tick-borne illnesses, we discovered that I had a few associated disorders like adrenal fatigue and a common triad found in Lyme patients: mast cell activation syndrome (MCAS), dysautonomia including postural orthostatic tachycardia syndrome (POTS), and hypermobile Ehlers-Danlos syndrome (hEDS). It didn't answer all of our questions, but it did give me some comfort. I was starting to see my symptoms for exactly what they were, and I felt a little less crazy as a result.

The lightning in my face was eventually identified as trigeminal neuralgia (TN). A rare, neurological condition causing severe electric-shock-type facial pain that has been described by the American Association of Neurological Surgeons as the "most excruciating pain known to humanity."

Talk about validating.

In fact, the only thing scientifically rated more painful than TN is another rare neurological condition called complex regional pain syndrome (CRPS). It is considered to be the "most excruciating *chronic* pain condition known," ranked more painful than unprepared childbirth and more painful than an amputation without anesthesia.

But then, it was only a few weeks later, with no better explanation for the attacks in my chest, that one of my new doctors concluded I had *that* as well. I had both of the top two worst pain conditions known. Naming them had *not* brought me the sense of relief that I'd all along dreamed it would.

I quickly learned that there was no cure and limited effective treatments for either TN or CRPS. For this, both had been nicknamed suicide diseases. A name was just a name in the end, no more helpful than the umbrella term "pain" if the doctors didn't know how to resolve it—and they didn't. After all of that time, still, no one had any idea how to help me.

I met with more doctors and scheduled more tests, filling my calendar with appointments, filling my calendar with hope. There was testing in neuro-ophthalmology and neurology, testing of my senses, reflexes, coordination, balance, and strength. There were studies of my brain and central nervous system, bloodwork every few days, EMG and nerve conduction testing, biopsies, and up to two-and-a-half hours in the MRI machine each time.

When finally, in June of 2021, doctor-number-twelve—my new Lyme-literate neurologist, Dr. Anne—diagnosed me with relapsing and remitting multiple sclerosis (MS).

"The pattern of demyelination is textbook for MS," she told me. "You most definitely have MS and have had it for some time."

For a second, but only a second, I questioned everything.

I knew I fit all the risk factors. I was genetically predisposed to autoimmune disease due to a family history. I was from the prairie provinces of Canada, which have one of the highest prevalences of MS in the entire world. I was female, of the right age, of Scandinavian descent, and I had low vitamin D and a complicated history with mononucleosis. Plus, I had every single symptom of the disease and the central nervous system lesions to prove it.

MS fit. And at that realization, I was immediately tempted to delete this entire book. This book about Lyme disease. Yet I sensed, somehow, that fit, too.

Lyme was often called "the great imitator," as it could mimic a number of autoimmune diseases, but I'd been learning it could also trigger them. New research showed that if left untreated for too long, *Borrelia burgdorferi* could indeed compromise the immune system and trigger multiple sclerosis—exactly what Dr. Anne believed happened to me.

She went on to confirm that they were absolutely two separate diseases, and I had them both. MS was the name for *what* was happening inside my body—and Lyme disease explained *why*.

In a way, we were all right.

I had Lyme disease. I'd always had Lyme disease. And I also had something else.

I accepted it—without fear, or pause, or anything. That explanation was the first thing in all of this that had immediately made sense to me. Instinctually, I knew it fit. I not only found it validating but liberating to have another piece of the puzzle click into place.

I continued to work with Dr. Anne all through that summer, and in October, she also diagnosed me with autoimmune small fiber peripheral neuropathy (SFN). My results showed that I was in the one percentile for nerve function at thirty-seven years old (testing even worse than most ninety-year-olds), yet I wasn't surprised by that either. I accepted it, too.

MS was in my central nervous system, and SFN was in my peripheral—I was being attacked from all angles. But of course I'd sensed that all along, it was only the names that were new to me.

I felt hopeful, armed with all of that new information. However, the hope that came with receiving those answers was dashed, yet again, when I learned that most MS and SFN treatments were going to be contraindicated because I also had Lyme. Again, I had a few more diagnoses, a few more names and explanations, but zero answers. I was denied five times in a row for the only treatment advised for all three diseases, intravenous immunoglobulin therapy (IVIG). I was left with no answers, no hope, and no treatment for my specific mix of illnesses.

Dr. Ryan, ironically, the same Lyme-guy I'd feared all along would leave me, ended up staying with me through this. We continued to meet precisely every four weeks, testing the theory that my Lyme was the root cause of the MS and the SFN, the adrenal fatigue, the MCAS, the POTS, the TN, and even the CRPS.

It was another theory I wasn't sure I could trust, but treating this hypothetical trigger felt like my only hope.

I spent my days tracking symptoms. Taking note of which symptoms Herxed and abated in response to which drugs, I was desperate to sort out which symptoms could be caused by pathogens. And seeing this, Dr. Ryan started to compliment my methods—learning to trust me and I him. I started to feel more in control of my health as I told him what had worked, what hadn't, and what prescriptions I would need more of—and he followed my lead.

Again I found myself surrounded by papers—charts and lists and printed research articles. But after another year with diligent tracking, I finally felt that some progress was being made. Together, Dr. Ryan and I were proving that my chronic Lyme was indeed a persistent infection, as we watched my symptoms respond directly to the antibiotic treatment that many old-school doctors would have never condoned.

I was finding some success with Krintafel, a drug Dr. Ryan had been experimenting with in his practice for *Babesia*. I'd been fearful to try the single-dose cure for malaria, but I ended up taking it a total of nineteen times—sometimes as often as every ten days, to keep my symptoms at bay. And as a result, the electrocutions in my chest started to fade away.

Methylene blue was proving to be the miracle drug for my *Bartonella*, the same way that Krintafel was for my *Babesia*. With it, the electrocutions of type I trigeminal neuralgia became fewer and farther in between until the attacks stopped altogether.

As for *Borrelia*, in the spring of 2022, I joined the five percent of Lyme patients who get treated with intravenous antibiotics when I had a PICC line surgically installed in my upper arm. It was fed inside my vein all the way up to my heart so that I could receive IV ceftriaxone twice daily.

I Herxed hard with that one, the pain of the Herxes in my chest particularly excruciating. I was completely bedridden and fading in and out of consciousness, unaware of the passage of time, day or night. I was certain the violent chest pain and arrhythmias were soon going to kill me. It seemed my body was once again shutting down.

The muscles in my arm spasmed violently, incessantly, as my body tried to reject the line. I started to develop blood clots. While on top of it all, due to the MCAS, I was allergic to the sterile dressing, the special chlorhexidine cleanser, and the ceftriaxone itself. Twice a day, while Marty administered my IV, I sneezed so forcefully I pulled chest muscles and leaked tears and snot everywhere.

Still, I persisted. I took about a dozen other drugs along with the IV ceftriaxone at that time, and it felt like a dangerous combination. But I knew something was starting to happen when the odor in my left arm suddenly changed, and my scalp erupted into a painful, itchy helmet of pustules that no doctor could figure out.

After two months of that, I felt the lights turn back on as I came back into consciousness. And another month later, my neck pain, which had been incapacitating for so incredibly long, vanished overnight. I rose to standing. It wasn't long after that when I started to drive again, walk with a cane, and, for the first time ever, I even managed to attend an appointment with Dr. Ryan all on my own.

In my hand, I held a list. All of my symptoms finally divided into three separate categories, three separate causes: *Borrelia*, *Babesia*, and *Bartonella*.

It appeared I had emerged on the other side.

"Whoa," Dr. Ryan said as a way of greeting me when I entered his office.

I smirked as I sat down in the familiar brown leather chair opposite his desk and set my cane and Fendi bag on the chair Marty usually occupied.

"Did you drive yourself here?"

"Yes," I laughed through my MAGO. My jaw was still sore, but at least I had some functionality back. "I do know how to drive, you know."

Dr. Ryan laughed, too. "Yes, yes, of course. I'm sure you do. Where is your husband, though? You've never once come alone."

"Today is also a big day for him," I replied, proudly. "He's selling his company." I handed Dr. Ryan my typed notes, ending the pleasantries there.

I needed to protect my still-dislocated jaw as much as possible, so I kept with our regular routine. I allowed Dr. Ryan to read the notes aloud while I waited silently. When he was done, we made our way to his testing table where I lay down and let my mind wander, staring up at those dingy ceiling tiles while he got to work. And twenty minutes later, we sat back at the mahogany desk where Dr. Ryan gave me the verdict.

"I'm glad to see you're doing better. I think, at this point, we've exhausted the PICC line's usefulness. I'm going to order to have it removed."

I wasn't sure if I was pleased with that decision or not. It had been in for four months at that point, the longest of any of his previous patients. And it had cost me $1,200 a week after insurance ($20,000 for the whole sixteen weeks). One-fifth of the total $100,000 I'd already spent to date. It hadn't been cheap, *and* it had almost killed me—yet I still thought it had been worth it. I estimated I was about fifty percent improved, and I craved so much more.

"At this point, it's just no longer worth the risk," Dr. Ryan continued. "And I'm going to send you next door for another ultrasound on that swollen arm. We need to check you for blood clots again, too."

I could see he was already starting to write out the order, so I let my mind wander to what would be next for me. I wondered what, if anything, he would be prescribing.

I'd grown tired of requiring dangerous drugs, and I feared needing them for the rest of my life. I'd heard about a clinic that did things differently—first from my dental surgeon, then on a podcast, and even from Dr. Ryan himself, who'd had a few former patients go there.

I was definitely interested.

I'd had enough of hearing Dr. Ryan say he'd already used all of his biggest guns on me. That the great majority of Lyme patients never even need the heavy-hitting drugs that I'd been on. Yet even with all that he'd given me, I was still testing quite poorly.

I was hoping that this month would be different, but he looked up from his writing and handed me a prescription. "Nine scripts for this month."

My heart sank as I automatically took the piece of paper from his outstretched hand, glancing down to see it was all the same stuff. Another month, more of the same. "How long are we supposed to do this for?"

"I don't know," he replied frankly. "I don't know why your immune system isn't kicking in. You're still very far from well. Probably in the worst, I don't know, three percent of my patients. One of the worst I've ever seen, honestly." He paused as if gathering himself. "But you haven't died yet."

He gave a small shrug as the word "yet" hung awkwardly in the air between us. We'd been pretty open with each other these days, but I still couldn't believe he'd actually said it. I'd always wondered if he understood how perilously close I'd been, not always trusting myself as an accurate narrator during the worst of those times. But his words told me that he had known. He was the doctor testing me each month, altering my medications as needed, and calling me in a panic whenever my bloodwork was off. This was just the first time he'd said it aloud.

I hadn't died yet.

I gathered my belongings, a bit stunned. I was serious about trying the alternative immunotherapy treatment I'd been hearing about, but I knew that if I did choose that path, I'd be choosing to leave Dr. Ryan for good. The two methods were contraindicated; I couldn't do both.

I was scared to leave him, scared to regress. We'd come a long way, he and I, and I'd really grown to trust him over the course of thirty straight months. But I felt that Dr. Ryan's own words had just somehow validated that I *should* be trying something else. After two-and-a-half years of aggressive treatments, he was still describing me as one of his worst patients. And still very far from well.

I paused at the doorway and turned back to face him. "Thank you," I said, looking Dr. Ryan directly in the eye. "For everything." And then I walked out with my nine repeat prescriptions, unsure if I would ever see him again.

I didn't know if I'd be an idiot to continue to take his medications. Or an idiot not to.

I spent that weekend pondering my options and reflecting on past choices. It occurred to me that I'd always been a bit of a follower, a people pleaser, often taking the path of least resistance and doing what others expected of me. I'd even started to suspect that I'd lost my voice a long time ago—long before my jaw ever dislocated.

It was well before the years when I let the doctors tell me I was "fine." Before I sat idly by and let Charlene verbally abuse the staff, and before I let the sparkle of the corporate world intimidate me into silence. I suspected it was even before all the years during which I ignored my own symptoms and pretended I was perfect. Before I followed my husband's career around to different cities. Or agreed to dates to spare boys' feelings. It was even before I sat mutely in the dance studio, intimidated by the older girls, and went to school dressed exactly like my sister.

I'd lost my voice a long time ago.

Or maybe, maybe I'd never really found it.

In an unexpected burst, I broke away from my people-pleasing tendencies then. Freeing myself from a lifetime performance of politeness, I left my biological TMJ specialist, Dr. Kim, as well as my now-trusted Lyme-guy, Dr. Ryan, behind. It was a sign of the newfound hope I was feeling, but also a sign that I was fed up. Gone were any straggling beliefs that anyone was going to come save me, least of all the Western medical system. I found my own voice among all the noise that surrounded me, as I chose to take the path less traveled by trying the alternative immunotherapy with doctor-number-eighteen.

For years, desperate people had been flying from all over the world to the small lake town of Coeur d'Alene, Idaho—all in the hope of seeing a doctor who'd nearly had his license revoked for attempting to cure Lyme patients with magnets.

It sounded impossible. Yet everything I'd read told me he'd been having some miraculous success.

Afraid to hope but perhaps more afraid not to, in September 2022, for the first time in three years, I got on a plane. Ready for it to be my time.

I was done with being sick. I'd put in the time, the money, the medications, and I was over it. I hadn't chosen this illness—the pain, the depression, or the psychosis. None of that had been my fault. I would always hate that I had Lyme disease—but I recognized that fighting it hadn't been getting me anywhere. I couldn't change what had happened to me or how I'd handled it in the past. I could only control what I chose next.

I let it all go.

I stopped projecting my pain onto poor Marty, realizing that I'd been stuck in the minutiae and missing the bigger picture. Overcome with gratitude that he had stayed when so many others would have chosen to leave, I saw that he had been showing his love for me through his actions all along.

He'd worked long days and then picked up the slack at home: cooking, cleaning, and caring for me. He'd bathed me when I could no longer care for myself and tenderly washed my hair. Administered my IVs twice a day and attended all of my appointments. He'd even moved back upstairs, falling into a bedroom routine of holding me in his arms and gently rubbing my back until we both fell asleep intertwined.

He'd picked me up whenever I fell, carried me when I couldn't walk, and held me as I'd cried, day after day. He'd stayed strong when I was weak and held onto hope when I had none. He'd shown me the true meaning of love, steady and strong, unwavering and unconditional.

Our hardest years had been some of our most beautiful.

They'd bonded us closer than we'd ever been.

I then unfollowed every sad, sick Instagram account that I'd once related to, and traded podcasts and books about sickness for ones about healing. I signed up for yet another neuroplasticity brain retraining program online, meditated, and focused on my wellness, visualizing a future for myself that didn't include anything medical.

I stopped saving empty pill bottles and threw away the near thousand I'd already collected like some perverse badge of honor. And I chose to stop adding up the financial costs of having Lyme disease, deciding that investing in my health with treatments wasn't much different from buying vitamins or healthy groceries.

I was moving on—accepting life for all that it was and wasn't. It may not have been the life I'd imagined or the life I would have chosen, but it was the life I had been given. So I chose to feel happiness and gratitude for what I could do in each moment rather than resentment for what I couldn't.

I tore down the Post-it notes that filled my walls with symptoms and clues and replaced them with joyful, positive, healing affirmations instead. I'd been learning that when we think negatively, every cell in our body can hear us—but I suspected it was more than that. The opposite could be true as well. Not only could our negative thoughts harm us, our positive thoughts could heal us.

I made the choice to be all in. I didn't just choose to believe in the new magnetic immunotherapy treatment; I believed in my body's own ability to heal itself, too. I started to visualize that my every action was doing just that.

It was slow.

And I was slow.

Though my pace was intentional this time. No longer feeling the need to keep up with the high speed of the world around me, I wondered when it was that our society had decided that busyness should be synonymous with success. And where did happiness fall into that equation, anyway? I made the conscious decision not to participate. Embracing my slower pace, I decided I was done with comparing.

I let go of the hurt I'd been holding onto—the hurt that had been caused when so many had let me down. Not necessarily forgetting it all —not yet—but forgiving. And maybe most importantly, I was reevaluating.

I'd always seen other people as so much more than me. So much greater. Placing them on a pedestal of assumed perfection and placing myself in an entirely different category. A category of much lesser value. It hadn't been fair—not to them or me. I'd inadvertently put too much pressure on them and expected too much, only ever succeeding in setting myself up for disappointment. I'd allowed them to hurt me, giving them a power over my feelings and sense of self-worth when that power should have only been mine.

With their hurt, they'd reminded me that they were just human, each with their own strengths and weaknesses, maybe not so different from me after all. No one was perfect in all areas—not even my family was. Yet I knew instinctively that discovering their imperfection would never cause me to love them any less. And it occurred to me that I probably should've been extending that same grace to myself all along.

If the people I had held in the highest regard weren't perfect, maybe I didn't need to be either.

So, along with the hurt, I let go of my competitiveness and my obsessive perfectionist tendencies, understanding once and for all that perfection was a myth. It was both subjective and a moving target, and basing my happiness or value on it had only ever been self-destructive.

I challenged myself to discover, and even embrace, my true, authentic self moving forward. For once, not with the goal of perfection, but to find my own unique value—sensitivity, insecurities, flaws, and all. And not in comparison to my sister. Or my husband. Or our friends, or anyone else. Just me, on my own.

And I think when I chose to let go of my perfectionism, I was choosing to be free.

I still had symptoms, I was still sick, but I didn't see myself that way anymore. I saw myself as healing as I burst from the metaphorical prison in which my mind had been keeping me trapped. I knew I was moving forward, even if it was at a turtle's speed. Forward was forward, I reminded myself. My speed didn't matter.

I stopped journaling about being sick and sad and lonely, and started to write about my healing and growth. Planning for the future for the first time in years, I researched hikes that I was determined I would someday take.

I'd come back to myself. The attitude, the grit, the athlete's mindset. The immediate retort that had always existed in the back of my mind on ready, but now I wasn't afraid to say aloud:

"Don't tell me what I can't do."

I told everyone around me that I was curing Lyme. Curing small fiber peripheral neuropathy. Curing multiple sclerosis. Accepting those diagnoses had been an important first step for me, but finally, I believed, truly believed in the depths of my soul, that I could heal from them. I was no longer striving for remission but instead a cure, and at times, my excitement and my hope were so clear in my mind that I questioned if I was having a manic break.

I wasn't.

I simply believed.

Eleven months later, in July of 2023, we traveled up to the Canadian Rockies to join my family in celebration as I turned forty years old.

Through the forest and among the dramatic jagged rock cliffs, I hiked to see the elusive emerald green of Lake Bourgeau and scrambled over Harvey Pass. It may have been rated as a hard fifteen miles with its forty-four hundred feet of elevation gain, but for me, as I climbed step after step, there was only an overwhelming sense of joy.

"Aim," Marty called from behind me. "You're killing me."

I turned around on the trail to see him—in his blue gym shorts and navy zip-up, with his hat on backward as usual. He was bent over with his hands on his knees and panting comically hard. I laughed.

"Sorry, babe!" I called back as I jogged easily down the trail a few yards to join him. Oh, how far we had come. I didn't even want to rest; with the endorphins pumping through me, I saw another peak in the distance, and I wanted to summit that, too. But I looked at my Marty then—my sweet, sweet Marty who was literally climbing mountains for me—and I happily sat on the rock beside him, letting my cane-turned-trekking-pole fall to the ground.

We rested there, side by side, in an alpine meadow, in a bowl near the top, with bighorn sheep, ptarmigan, and hoary marmots all around. The sun was warm, yet the slight breeze was cool on our skin, and the sky was a near-perfect clear blue. With only the odd marshmallowy, pure white puff of cloud hanging about, our proximity at that altitude gave the illusion we could reach out a hand and plunge it straight into their softness.

There were no bugs, no flies, not even mosquitoes. It was perfect. Silent and still, save for the call of the odd songbird off in the distance. And as we looked out at the breathtaking vista of the mountain peaks that make up the Continental Divide, my eyes followed a meandering creek down to the lake and sheer rock walls of the glacially carved amphitheater where we'd passed through below. The vast forest where we'd started was a pure, uninterrupted color block of dark evergreens, well beyond it all.

I reflected in soundless serenity, taking it all in.

The magnificence of my surroundings, the beauty of our love, and the magnitude of my accomplishment.

The very next day, we hiked an easy seven miles, my heart swelling, captivated by the mesmerizing electric blue of Moraine Lake. And the day after that, we hiked the Big Beehive, again rated as hard—stretching on for ten miles and rising twenty-four hundred feet above the awe-inspiring turquoise-colored waters of Lake Louise. The grand château where we'd started now so minuscule in the distance.

Next, we hiked eleven miles and fifteen hundred feet of elevation to the top of Thompson Falls with JJ. We hung our heads over the roar of the punchbowl to see the minty-aqua-colored water carve its way through the limestone of the slot canyon. Then it was six miles through the forest around two Cedar Lakes, where we swam in the waters as a family with our mom and dad. And finally, an exhilarating seven miles took us up above the treeline to summit both of the Terminator Peaks on Kicking Horse Mountain.

I was in remission.

I was alive.

THE BEGINNING OF ANOTHER

I found a life after Lyme, but even more importantly, I found myself. I simply had to keep fighting for it.

 I believe it was the combined effect of it all that saved me. Whether I felt any positive outcome from a specific treatment or therapy at the time or not, I don't consider any of it to have been a waste of my time, energy, or money. The treatments for the physical infections—pharmaceuticals, homeopathy, herbs, and supplements—all chipped away at the infections. While restorative health practices, detoxification, and a dedication to clean living helped lower the overall toxicity in my metaphorical soup pot. I honored the mind-body connection, surrounded myself with the right people—was unconditionally loved and supported by those people—and intentionally chose to live a more stress-free, loving life. And finally, there were four trips to the magnet-man in Idaho to boost my immune system and get me over the finish line.

 There have been a few bumps in the road since then, of course. After achieving remission in the summer of 2023, I relapsed only a few months later. I had to learn to accept that—the ebbs and the flows. Neither life nor Lyme is as black and white as I once hoped. And chronic illness is just that—there really isn't an end.

This likely finds me somewhere in the middle, the middle of a lifelong journey. My times with the Lyme-guy (doctor-number-ten) and the magnet-man (doctor-number-eighteen) were only just the beginning. Over the last five years, I've now sought help from a staggering forty-one doctors (and counting).

My life looks a little different now, different from what I ever imagined. I don't get to go back to how I was before, not after surviving an illness like this. I've had to accept that, too. But I choose to take it one day at a time, and I try to see the lessons and the growth instead of focusing on the pain.

I see my illness, not unlike the leaves in the fall, as an indication of changing seasons. And I believe beauty can be found there—in the liminal space—sometimes we just have to look a little bit harder for it. My brief time hiking in the majestic Canadian Rockies has inspired me to continue. I believe I'm on the precipice of another remission, my time soon coming. I just have to keep going for a little while longer.

With my illnesses mostly manageable, I've turned my focus onto healing the damages that occurred as a result. The doctors believe that the trigeminal neuralgia was the source of the violent muscle spasm that dislocated my jaw. But as for why it's not healed yet—well, every doctor has had a different theory on that.

Some have described it as a bandwidth issue, a breakdown of the processing power. They say my body cannot compute information at the necessary level of refinement for the dislocation to heal. Spasticity or tone from the MS has been presumed to be trapped, preventing the jaw displacement from relaxing and realigning. Others have been more blunt, hypothesizing that my trigeminal nerve has been fried and my jaw will never work correctly again. Some believe the root cause is in my neck. A few even believe that I must have always had a dysfunctional, though asymptomatic, jaw—a predisposition due to my hypermobility, a laxity in the joint. They were even so bold to say that the dislocation had been inevitable all along. But the one thing all the doctors have agreed on is that there isn't a surgery that can fix this.

I'm working with dentist-number-fifteen now, a physiologic dentist accredited in TMJD through the Las Vegas Institute. Dr. Scott treats me with transcutaneous electric nerve stimulation, ultrasound, and cold, low-level lasers, as well as with two new orthotics. He hooks me up to an EMG machine every two weeks to assess the functionality of my muscles and nerves, while a T-Scan determines the location, force, and timing of my bite—all the fundamental parameters for measuring occlusion. It's very scientific.

Yet I think the most interesting thing Dr. Scott offers me is manual manipulation.

At six foot four and easily two hundred fifty pounds, Dr. Scott stands facing me. He places his thumbs into my mouth and onto my lower molars as he wraps the rest of his fingers under my mandible, gripping my face. And then he pulls. He moves my jaw. Manipulates it. He feels for the resistance of my muscles, ligaments, and tendons—he stretches them, attempting to coax my discs and condyles back into their proper positions. All the while, I grip the arms of the dental chair, resisting the tears that threaten to run down my cheeks.

I'm hopeful—even if it has been five years and my teeth still do not occlude. Without an orthotic in my mouth, I have zero ability to chew. And I do still suffer from some bilateral type II trigeminal neuralgia, as well as the occasional type I, which prevents me from working or socializing.

I know I've got a ways to go. And I'm not really sure what's next for me.

Will I be able to achieve remission again?

Will my jaw ever heal?

Is Lyme disease ever fully gone?

And will I be able to keep the MS from progressing?

I don't know. And I'm going to have to be okay with that, because there will always be more unknowns than knowns in life. Accepting that enormity is perhaps the greatest lesson I will come to learn.

An absolute acceptance. I do think I'm on my way.

Life isn't fair, often doesn't make sense, and we have very little control over any of it. And no life, no career, marriage, or human is perfect. There is only trying. There are only lessons. And life, like Lyme, is one big, painful lesson.

I've been learning to accept it all. Life, Lyme, and myself. Recognizing that even as I strive to become a better version of myself, there can't always be "delicate blossoming. You will become, and unbecome. And there will be sun, and there will be storm."[4]

I've even come to accept that while I may have fought Lyme disease for thirty-one years, I no longer believe I lost even a single day to it. This disease is a part of my journey.

And it's only one segment. One chapter. One season (even if it did feel like a long one). One snapshot of who I was in a few moments of time—but those moments have already passed, and I'm already no longer that girl. It is one storyline of what will be many, interwoven with all the others that will eventually make up my life. It may be a part of my history, but Lyme will never define me. I am so much more than any single thing.

I am my mother's giant heart and my father's sense of humor. A little girl awed by nature, imagining a world among the lily pads. And even when all grown up, a girl who will always see the magic.

I hold inside my heart laughter with friends, the love of my family, and Pete's wagging tail. The serenity of healing walks with JJ and the look in Marty's eye when we first professed our love. The squeaking sounds of sneakers on a basketball court, the hoofbeats of galloping horses, and the echoes of children weeping on the steps of St. Joseph's church.

I am mountains climbed and countries moved. The cool ripples of a lake and a hurricane alike. I am art and I am design, grief and love, and emotion, for which words will never be enough.

I am all of these things and more, shaped by all of my life experiences. My wins and losses alike, and everything in between.

Constantly evolving. My future unknown.

I am me, and I am still becoming.

APPENDIX I

WORKING LIST OF SYMPTOMS AND DIAGNOSES,
compiled 2019–2022:

1. C3-C4: uncovertebral joint hypertrophy with neural foraminal narrowing, **painful to the touch**.
2. L4-L5: disc bulge shallow protrusion.
3. L5-S1: spondylolysis, anterolisthesis, unroofing of disc margin and bulging.
4. T10-T11: spinal canal narrowing, disc at loss and osteophyte formation, **extremely painful to the touch**.
5. ABDOMEN: **debilitatingly sharp** pain in lower right quadrant, refers through to back, worse after urinating, intense localized pain by belly button (specifically at eleven o'clock), diagonal line of fire from side ribs to pubic bone, causes to **remain doubled over**.
6. ADRENAL FATIGUE: **orthostatic intolerance**, low blood pressure, digestive issues, arrhythmias, hair loss, fatigue, insomnia (specifically waking up between two and four a.m.), **overwhelm** and difficulty coping with stress, **brain fog**, pain in upper back and neck, difficulty remembering, overemotionality, irritability, depression, anxiety, feeling cold, sensitivity to light, salt cravings, easily startled and can't calm down after, food intolerances, environmental allergies.
7. AGORAPHOBIA: complete **inability to leave safe space** for fear of panic and embarrassment.
8. ANEMIA
9. ASTHENIA: loss of strength, loss of vitality, doctor suggested a diagnosis of myasthenia gravis (MG).
10. BEAU'S LINES: sudden onset of horizontal lines on fingernails, indicating a health event.
11. BLADDER: urge **incontinence**, frequent urination, pain in LRQ of abdomen, suggested diagnoses of interstitial cystitis or pelvic floor dysfunction.
12. BRAIN: **lesions** in white matter, **T2 flair hyperintensities**, **T1 hypointensities**, encephalitis, increased intracranial pressure, encephalopathy.
13. BREASTS: swelling, aching pain, and sensitivity.
14. CALF (RIGHT): constant cramp, pressure, vice-like tightness, numbness.
15. CANDIDA: reoccurring oral thrush, parageusia/dysgeusia (persis-

tent metallic taste in mouth).
16. CARDIAC: **heart attack-like pain, arrhythmias, tachycardia**, atrial fibrillation, murmur.
17. CELIAC DISEASE: ten plus years of **chronic diarrhea** prior to diagnosis, bloating, food sensitivities and intolerances.
18. CENTRAL SENSITIZATION: allodynia (pain to non-noxious stimuli), hyperalgesia (increased sensitivity to pain), sensory hyperarousal, **misophonia** (extreme sensitivity to noise), **photophobia** (extreme eye sensitivity to light), **hyperosmia** (extreme sensitivity to smell), misokinesia (extreme sensitivity to movements), **hyperacusis** (extreme sensitivity to sounds resulting in physical pain).
19. COGNITIVE DYSREGULATION: extreme, all or nothing thinking, **paranoia**, dissociative responses, cognitive blackouts, **personality changes**.
20. COGNITIVE IMPAIRMENT: **confusion**, brain fog, deteriorated concentration/focus/comprehension/association/processing speed/word finding/communication/memory, impaired sleep, getting lost in own home, inability to recognize faces of family members, **personality changes**.
21. COMPLEX POST TRAUMATIC STRESS DISORDER (CPTSD): dysregulation, trapped in **fight-or-flight**, intrusive thoughts, distrust, avoidance, depression, and suicidal ideation resulting from prolonged, repeating medical trauma.
22. COMPLEX REGIONAL PAIN SYNDROME (CRPS): levels 8, 9, and 10 pain, **blackouts**.
23. COUGH: dry, usually in the middle of the night.
24. LONG COVID
25. DEPRESSION: emotional dysregulation, major clinical episodes, dysthymia, **suicidal ideation**.
26. DISSOCIATION: derealization, detachment, depersonalization, micro-amnesias.
27. DYSAUTONOMIA: noise/light sensitivity, **shortness of breath**, **dizziness**, vertigo, temperature dysregulation, tachycardia, arrhythmias, brain fog, mood swings, **orthostatic intolerance**, syncope, nausea, inability to sweat, sleep disturbances, bladder incontinence.
28. ELBOW (LEFT): constant throb in joint, numbness down forearm and into fingers.
29. EMOTIONAL DYSREGULATION: inability to manage emotional responses, resulting in **psychosis**, needing to reduce or escape emotions by not managing them through **dissociation**/derealization/detachment/depersonalization/micro-amnesias, amygdala hi-

jack/fight-or-flight, mood swings/irritability/outbursts/anger, anxiety, depression, personality changes.
30. ENCEPHALOMYELITIS
31. ENDOMETRIOSIS: **chronic abdominal pain**, worse after urinating (dysuria), unusually light periods, excessive menstrual cramping (dysmenorrhea).
32. EPSTEIN BARR VIRUS
33. EYES/VISION: sudden onset of **pressure, floaters, and blurriness** in right eye (exacerbated by heat), sharp stinging pain, alternating cold and burning sensations in left eye, symmetric thinning/loss of papillomacular bundle consistent with demyelinating disease, **optic neuritis** (ON), bilateral demyelinating inflammation of the optic nerves, subclinical/asymptomatic ON in the left eye, ON in right eye with atypical duration, hallucinations/peripheral vision disturbances.
34. EXHAUSTION: **extreme fatigue**, lethargy, lassitude.
35. FASCICULATIONS: incessant muscle twitching, single muscle twitch can last for months at a time.
36. FEAR: intrusive ruminating thoughts, stuck in **fight-or-flight** mode.
37. FEET: plantar fasciitis, **debilitating pain in soles** that prevents walking or standing, paresthesias (**numbness** and tingling in heels, **burning toes**, sensation of all toes being broken, sensation of walking on broken glass, skin intensely painful to the touch, pressure in right big toenail, webbing feels torn between fourth and fifth toes), swollen arthritic joints.
38. FINGERS: paresthesia (**numbness** and burning), arthralgia.
39. GABA DEFICIENCY
40. GAIT: drop foot, inability to lift legs high enough to properly walk, **ataxia**, loss of balance, coordination, loss of motor control, weakness and buckling, stiffness, rigidity, spasticity, all resulting in **inability to walk**.
41. GENERALIZED ANXIETY DISORDER
42. HAIR: significant episodes of hair loss, sudden change in color.
43. HYPERMOBILE EHLERS-DANLOS SYNDROME (hEDS/hypermobility spectrum disorder): hypermobility causing a genetic predisposition/susceptibility to both the adverse effects of tick-borne illness and potential root of TMJ dislocation.
44. HYPERTENSION: periodic.
45. HYPOTENSION: chronic, **dizziness**, **syncope**, vision changes, weakness.
46. HYPOTHYROIDISM: weight gain, weight loss.
47. INSOMNIA: difficulty falling asleep, difficulty staying asleep, and

difficulty falling back asleep once woken.
48. JAUNDICE: periodic.
49. KIDNEYS: aching throb, sensitivity to touch.
50. KNEES: both knees arthritic, right knee cracks, pops, and grinds, sharp pain in left kneecap.
51. LEAKY GUT
52. LIMBIC SEIZURES
53. LIVER: discomfort, inflammation.
54. LUMBAR: sharp, seizing, at times aching.
55. LYME DISEASE: **tick-borne illness** including, but not limited to ***Borrelia burgdorferi***, *Borrelia recurrentis, Babesia divergens, Babesia duncani, Bartonella henselae, Mycoplasma pneumoniae.*
56. MAST CELL ACTIVATION SYNDROME (MCAS): **extreme allergy attacks** presenting as chronic diarrhea, full body rashes, rash on arms, rash on legs, perioral dermatitis, keratosis pilaris, lip swelling and tingling.
57. MERALGIA PARESTHETICA (MP): paresthesia, usually numb, yet at times painful to the touch as if a piece of metal is embedded in flesh.
58. METHEMOGLOBINEMIA
59. MICROSCOPIC COLITIS: **re-onset of chronic diarrhea** despite following Celiac diet, intolerance to sugar.
60. MOLD ILLNESS/MYCOTOXINS
61. MOTION SICKNESS: **extreme and progressive**, preventing almost all vehicular travel.
62. MULTIPLE AUTOIMMUNE SYNDROME (MAS): diagnosed as **three or more distinct autoimmune conditions** (celiac, multiple sclerosis, small fiber peripheral neuropathy, microscopic colitis).
63. MULTIPLE SCLEROSIS (MS): **demyelinating nerve damage** resulting in **disrupted communication throughout body**. Presenting as ataxia, drop foot, spasticity, bladder issues, numbness, tingling, burning, pain, MS hug, vision loss, optic neuritis, fatigue, tremor and internal tremor, dizziness, heat intolerance, mood disturbances, dysphagia, cognitive impairment.
64. MS HUG: **debilitating pain in celiac/solar plexus,** constricting pressure banding/girdling/**corset** that wraps around the lower ribs/upper abdomen/solar plexus, making it hard to eat, hard to breathe, often exacerbated by eating or contact with clothing.
65. MUSCLE SPASMS: **violent and uncontrollable**, resulting in bilateral TMJ dislocation.
66. NAUSEA: persistent.
67. NECK: **severe pinching pain** and stiffness, excessive crepitus,

APPENDIX I

      limited mobility.
68. NIGHT TERRORS
69. NOSEBLEEDS: severe and chronic.
70. OBSESSIVE COMPULSIVE DISORDER (OCD): intrusive ruminating **paranoias** leading to **illogical compulsions**, disrupts normal life.
71. OSTEOARTHRITIS/ARTHRALGIA: fingers and hands, right ankle, both knees, left hip, spine, jaw.
72. PANIC ATTACKS: sudden incapacitating **episodes of terror**, including **hyperventilating**, sobbing, shortness of breath, racing heart, dissociation, derealization.
73. PARASITES
74. PELVIS: incapacitating **internal electric shock** nerve pain attacks, aching bones that prevent sitting.
75. PIRIFORMIS SYNDROME: debilitating pain following length of piriformis muscle.
76. POST TRAUMATIC STRESS DISORDER (PTSD): anxiety and **flashbacks** of traumatic events, **avoidance** of triggers.
77. POSTURAL ORTHOSTATIC TACHYCARDIA SYNDROME (POTS): orthostatic hypotension, **orthostatic intolerance**, syncope, near-syncope, temperature dysregulation.
78. PSEUDOBULBAR AFFECT (PBA): random, **pathological**, uncontrollable crying without cause.
79. PSYCHOSIS: Lyme **psychosis**/rage, extreme dysregulation, loss of reality.
80. PULMONARY: asthma, **air hunger**, dyspnea (shortness of breath).
81. RAYNAUD'S SYNDROME: secondary Raynaud's phenomenon.
82. RIBS/CHEST: two distinct types of pain. Type I: **level 10** incapacitating sudden bursts of **electric shock** type neuropathic pain in ribs and sternum that radiate down arm and through to back, resulting in **blackouts**. Type II: level 8 incapacitating constant stabbing/tearing/**burning** pain in chest, ribs, sternum, and upper back, resulting in difficulty breathing, prevents sitting or lying down.
83. SELF DYSREGULATION: unstable sense of self and sense of **emptiness**.
84. SHOULDERS: bursitis, crunching noises and intense shooting nerve pains in scapula.
85. SINUS: blocked maxillary sinus, sharp pains, uncomfortable burning, dryness, shooting pains from nostril deep into head.
86. SKIN: **pustules** on scalp, acne around jaw, burnt rash, *Bartonella*

UNACCEPTABLE

rash, extreme sensitivity to touch and temperature, pruritus (neuropathic itch), crawling skin, easy bruising, unexplained body rashes, **perioral dermatitis**, keratosis pilaris.
87. SMALL FIBER PERIPHERAL NEUROPATHY (SFPN): polyneuropathy (**pain**, paresthesia, tingling/**numbness**/pins and needles/**burning**, orthostatic hypotension, difficulty adjusting eyes from light to dark, inability to sweat in lower legs and feet, bladder issues, dizziness and fainting, difficulty breathing, high heart rate, hypersensitivity).
88. SPASTICITY: rigidity preventing movement of limbs.
89. TAILBONE: debilitating pinching pain in coccyx, with referred ache.
90. TEMPORAL MANDIBULAR JOINT (TMJ): sudden and severe overnight bilateral **articular disc dislocation** and **subluxation/ dislocation of condyles** resulting in severe jaw misalignment/extreme open bite, capsulitis, trismus (**inability to open the mouth or jaw**), **inability to chew or speak**, muscle twitching and spasms, arthralgia, **constant facial migraine** including temporalis, neck, eyes, ears, and teeth, tinnitus.
91. THERMOREGULATION: poor ability to regulate body temperature, intolerance to hot or cold, **chills** dominant, body temperature readings of ninety-five degrees Fahrenheit, **drenching night sweats**, cold triggers spasticity and tremor.
92. THIGH (LEFT): deep, boring **neurogenic pain**.
93. THROAT/TRACHEA: sharp shooting pains, intermittent closing, **dysphagia** (difficulty swallowing), odynophagia (painful swallowing), **globus sensation** (sensation of choking).
94. TREMOR (EXTERNAL): visibly starts in right hand, takes over entire body, triggered by stress, exacerbated by cold.
95. TREMOR (INTERNAL): vibration/buzz felt in lower torso, not outwardly visible.
96. TRIGEMINAL NEURALGIA (TN): bilateral type I: extreme **electric shock nerve pain attacks** (like lightning bolts) predominantly through maxillary and ophthalmic branches. Atypical type II: **constant searing pain** in jaw, eyes, ears, and teeth. Occasional facial hypoesthesia (numbness or tingling) around eye and cheek.
97. VERTIGO: dizziness, spinning, sense of unstableness.
98. VITAMIN B12 DEFICIENCY
99. VITAMIN D DEFICIENCY

APPENDIX II

MCGILL PAIN INDEX—designed to provide quantitative measures of clinical pain,[5] allowing for direct comparison across conditions.

50

CRPS (46)
trigeminal neuralgia (44)
kidney stones (42)

40

amputation of a digit (39)

unprepared child birth (36)

prepared child birth (32) ankylosing spondylitis (32)

30

fibromyalgia (30)

chronic back pain (28)

non-terminal cancer (26)
phantom limb pain (25)

after shingles nerve pain (22) bruise (22)

20

toothache (19)
fracture (18) arthritis (18)
cut (17)

laceration (15)
sprain (14)

10

tension headache (11)

no pain (0)

REFERENCES

MY GRATITUDE to those who came before me—publishing information as information was exactly what I needed.

WORKS CITED

[1] Rawls, Dr William. *Unlocking Lyme: Myths, Truths, and Practical Solutions for Chronic Lyme Disease.* Vital Plan, Inc. 2017.
[2] Bennett-Henry, Stephanie. Facebook, April 22, 2018. https://www.facebook.com/photo/?fbid=2156432614638295&set=a.1415488082066089.
[3] Frankl, Viktor E. *Man's Search for Meaning.* Beacon Press, 1946.
[4] Al-Thibeh, Isra. "The Moon Is a Witness." Accessed November 21, 2017.
[5] Melzack, Ronald. "The McGill Pain Questionnaire: Major properties and scoring methods." The Journal of the International Association for the Study of Pain 1(3):p 277-299. September, 1975.

BIBLIOGRAPHY

American Association of Neurological Surgeons. "Trigeminal Neuralgia." Accessed April 25, 2021. https://www.aans.org/Patients/Neurosurgical-Conditions-and-Treatments/Trigeminal-Neuralgia.
Aron, Dr Elaine. *The Highly Sensitive Person.* Harmony, 1996.
Bay Area Lyme Foundation. October, 2020. https://www.bayarealyme.org.
Bransfield, Robert C. "Suicide and Lyme and Associated Diseases." Neuropsychiatric Disease and Treatment 13 (2017): 1575-1587. https://pubmed.ncbi.nlm.nih.gov/28670127/.
Caesar, Andrea H. *A Twist of Lyme: Battling a Disease That Doesn't Exist.* Archway Publishing, 2013.
"The History of Moose Jaw." Canada EHX. October 9, 2022. https://canadaehx.com/2022/10/09/the-history-of-moose-jaw/.
Centers for Disease Control and Prevention. October, 2020. https://www.cdc.gov.
Church, Lisa R. *Something's Wrong: When Life Gives You Lyme—What's Killing Me Could Be Killing You Too.* Resource Publications, 2019.
Cousins, Norman. Author of "Anatomy of an Illness." Accessed September 2, 2020 via Instagram (@heln83).
Crystal, Jennifer. Global Lyme Alliance. Accessed October, 2020. https://globallymealliance.org.

Douthat, Ross. The *Deep Places: A Memoir of Illness and Discovery*. Convergent Books, 2021.

Fallon, Brian A, MD, MPH, Trine Madsen, PhD, Annette Erlangsen, PhD, and Michael E Benros, MD, PhD. "Lyme Borreliosis and Associations With Mental Disorders and Suicidal Behavior: A Nationwide Danish Cohort Study," *American Journal of Psychiatry*, Volume 178, Number 10, 2021. https://doi.org/10.1176/appi.ajp.2021.200913.

Farnsworth, Vanessa. *Rain on a Distant Roof: A Personal Journey Through Lyme Disease in Canada*. Signature Editions, 2013.

"20 Root Causes of Inflammation." Accessed May 8, 2020 via Instagram (@funtional.foods_).

Global Lyme Alliance. October, 2020. https://globallymealliance.org.

"Lyme Disease Diagnosis: Key Steps in Diagnosing Lyme disease. Global Lyme Alliance. October, 2020. https://www.globallymealliance.org/about-lyme/diagnosis/.

Hilfiger, Ally. *Bite Me: How Lyme Disease Stole my Childhood, Made Me Crazy, and Almost Killed Me*. Center Street, 2016.

Hemingway, Ernest. *The Sun Also Rises*. Scribner, 1926.

"Lyme Innovation: Data-Driven, Patient-Centered Innovation for Tickborne Diseases." HealthData.gov. October, 2020. https://www.healthdata.gov.

International Lyme and Associated Diseases Society. October, 2020. https://www.ilads.org.

Kelland, Kate. "U.N. warns of mental health crisis due to COVID-19 pandemic." Reuters. May 14, 2020.

Khakpour, Porochista. *Sick: A Memoir*. Harper Collins, 2018.

Liu, Ming Di. "Who Am I?" *The Minds Journal*. Accessed September 24, 2017.

Lyme Warrior US. https://www.lymewarrior.us.

Naylor, Dr Shawn. "Chronic Infection: Lyme Disease." Sound Clinic. 2015. https://soundclinic.com/chronic-infection/lyme-disease/.

Project Lyme. https://www.projectlyme.org.

Reflex Sympathetic Dystrophy Syndrome Association. Accessed May 6, 2021. https://www.rsds.org.

Scher, Amy B. *This is How I Save My Life: From California to India, a True Story of Finding Everything When You Are Willing to Try Anything*. Gallery Books, 2018.

Spector, Dr Neil. "Lyme: The Infectious Disease Equivalent of Cancer, Says Top Duke Oncologist." HuffPost. February 19, 2016. https://www.huffpost.com/entry/lyme-the-infectious-disea_b_9243460.

"Spine Universe" and "Muncie Spine and Rehabilitation." September 26, 2020. https://spineuniverse.com; https://munciespine.com.

Strasheim, Connie. *New Paradigms in LYME DISEASE Treatment*. BioMed Publishing Group, 2016.

REFERENCES

The Lyme Times. Touched by Lyme. https://www.lymedisease.org.

The Tick Chicks. https://www.thetickchicks.com.

Tick Boot Camp. https://www.tickbootcamp.com.

Valpone, Amie. "The Trigger that Pops Your Balloon: What Activated Your Health Issues and Symptoms?" The Healthy Apple. May 9, 2017. https://healthyapple.com/the-trigger-that-pops-your-balloon-what-activated-your-health-issues-and-symptoms/.

Weintraub, Pamela. *Cure Unknown*. St. Martin's Griffin, 2009.

White, Emily Reach. Touched by Lyme. Accessed October, 2020. www.lymedisease.org.

www.ingramcontent.com/pod-product-compliance
Lightning Source LLC
Chambersburg PA
CBHW032101090426
42743CB00007B/196